Pathways to the Healing Arts Series
Volume 1

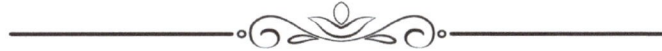

Become a Healing Arts Practitioner

A Map for Self-Healing
&
Manual for Certification

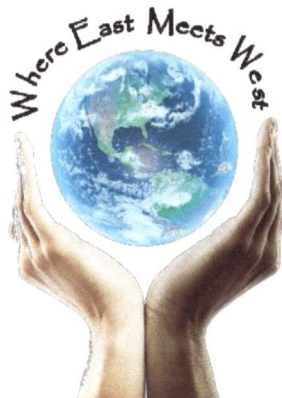

Joanne Kain Dinsmore
www.ClaremontHealingUSA.com

email: ClaremontHealingUSA@gmail.com
or ClaremontHealing@aol.com

Dedication

To
Mom and Dad
and our precious family tree.

What lies behind us and
what lies before us are
small matter compared to
what lies within us.

Ralph Waldo Emerson

Acknowledgements

Writing this book was ultimately and utmost a labor of love.

I am tremendously grateful for the significant spiritual teachers and mentors who awakened and guided me, whom have since passed on. Bless you all.

I am equally grateful for my parents, family, friends and clients who perhaps unknowingly have been my teachers and gifts from God.

The production and completion of this book would not have been possible without the graphic art skills of my friend and business partner, Julie Bradshaw. Many thanks, Jewels, for your endless patience, support and steadfast commitment to the mission.

I extend a great big hug of thanks to my photo models:

Alex (Snort) Hudspeth
(Julie's Grandson)

Karina Felix, HP, HHC

Katriana Walrath

George Maldonado, HP, HHC

Judy Ott-McGoon

Doug Dinsmore

And last but certainly not least, I thank my beloved editor and husband, Doug Dinsmore, for his dedication and unyielding support of my vision.

Dedication
Acknowledgements

Table of Contents

Editor's Foreword
Welcome to Volume One

Chapter 1: *The Healing Arts*

Chapter 2: *Self Growth & Discovery*

Chapter 3: *The Energy Fields*

Chapter 4: *Mind-Body Meditations*

Chapter 5: *Preparation for Healers*

Chapter 6: *The Healing Techniques*

Chapter 7: *The Shaman Path*

Chapter 8: *Healing With the Senses*

Chapter 9: *Conversing with Consciousness*

Chapter 10: *Certification Procedures*

Volume 2 The Road Continues

Editor's Foreword

The topics covered in this volume are considered by most students of the Western school of scientific thought to have no validity because of "unscientific" or seemingly "impossible" statements, such as the ability to heal by means of concentration of thought, or to detect illnesses by way of examination of auras.

Quantum Physics is a product of that same Western school of scientific thought, yet this field of "scientific" inquiry has produced many "impossible" declarations of its own, such as the assertion that an electron can occupy two different spaces simultaneously. The assertion continues with the condition that it only does so as long as it remains unobserved. Once observed, it occupies only a single space.

This implies that it is the act of observation which determines the electron's place in the physical universe. Observation is one aspect of thought. Thoughts are real. Thoughts are composed of something. Since thoughts have no physical form, then they must be composed of energy. Energy definitely has an effect on matter.

For example, in the Himalayan Mountains, there are Tibetan Buddhist monks who have been documented as being able to raise the temperature of their extremities by as much as 17 degrees F in sub-freezing weather, after being draped with wet towels. They managed to lower their metabolisms by as much as 60 percent at the same time, all through the power of their thoughts.

Semyon Davidovich Kirlian began taking photographs of people in 1939 which showed what he termed the human "aura", or energy field, which each human being projects continuously. Additionally, images taken using a Charged Coupled Device, an extremely sensitive piece of equipment, have depicted pictures of energy being exuded from the fingertips of healers. These are images of real energy, captured using proven scientific equipment and they have been used by healers for diagnosing various illnesses and disorders.

From these examples, it can be deduced that thoughts have some sort of influence on our bodies, as well as the physical universe. This being so (and quantum theory indicates that it is), then it should not be impossible for a healer to bring about healing through the concentration of thought. As a practicing healer, this author knows this to be true, for she has witnessed and produced the actual results outlined in the book many times.

The author seeks to enlighten the minds of the readers who choose to access the information provided in this book. She has attempted to do so in as factual a manner as possible. It is left to the reader to decide whether to accept the information thus offered or to reject it. The author asks only that the reader remember the cliché about minds: They are like parachutes- they only function when open.

Welcome to Volume One
in the Healing Arts Series

Many of the ideas and concepts covered in this book have been the subject of ridicule and outright rejection during the course of Western scientific history.

But you will find, as you read through it, that there are in fact sound scientific processes at work in many of them. Scientifically verifiable processes.

For example, brain wave activity can be altered by controlled breathing, muscle relaxation techniques and the changes measured and observed.

The physical and emotional benefits of meditation are discussed at some length in the book and are measurable and observable, as well.

If you can accept that everything that has been said so far is also believable, then you will be in the proper frame of mind to receive and experience the information provided within the pages of this book.

There are more things in Heaven and Earth, Horatio, than are dreamt of in your philosophy.
Hamlet, Act I, Scene V

Generally the healing arts are the field of study in holistic therapies to facilitate recovery and maintain balanced health for one's mind, body and spirit.

Because of the numerous sources of such natural methodologies, it is up to each of us to explore and discover which therapy or combination of therapies work best for us and our clients.

Our Pathways to the Healing Arts series offers you a wide range of practices to choose from in this growing field. After each sampling, we sincerely hope we've accomplished our goal in presenting a balanced approach for alternative and complimentary healing for body, mind and spirit.

Chapter 1

The Healing Arts

"Success in your work, the finding a better method, the better understanding that insures the better performing is hat and coat, is food and wine, is horse and health and holiday. At least, I find that any success in my work as the effect on my spirits of all these."

RALPH WALDO EMERSON

Introduction

What this book IS:

This manual is Part One of the healing series. It is designed for self-healing as well as an option for certification. A compilation over 30 years of my experience, it covers a broad range of topics and contains a considerable amount of information that no other single book has offered to date. My hope in gathering this information together in one place and presenting it to you is that those of you who are curious and find this text to be enlightening and insightful will be inspired to explore more thoroughly and eventually practice the healing arts.

We come from every walk of life; practice every religion and spiritual path. There are no prerequisites to become a healer except one: the desire to help others. This book will help you understand the ways of healing and what they're all about.

It is also an educational tool and reference. However, just reading the book alone is not enough to qualify you as a healer. It offers a solid and detailed foundation of knowledge that you can work with and practice to become an effective healing practitioner.

What this book is NOT:

This book is not a compilation of every healing method or style known. I have presented the core information found in many of the healing practices and techniques that I have learned over the years through my studies and personal discoveries. It begins with important basic information and progresses naturally into several healing modalities.

You will get out of it what you put into it and, like anything you work hard for, the rewards are invaluable.

How to use this book:

I strongly recommend that you follow this book from beginning to end. Each chapter builds on the last and gives you a "map", so to speak, to follow this journey wherever it may eventually take you. There are several exercises to help you practice what has been taught in the preceding chapter. You may want to read through the chapter, then go back and do the exercise(s). It is also a wonderful reference book to use in helping others understand the type of healing you're performing for and with them, as well as teaching them how to take greater responsibility in facilitating their own healing.

Know that, even after my 30 years of experience, I am still learning. The creation of this book alone has been a journey in and of itself. If you find a particular healing model that speaks to you more than another (i.e. reflexology vs. energy healing), please continue to explore it, learn it and share it. That's what it's all about! At the end of the book is the email address at which you may contact me with any questions, concerns or comments you may have.

Personal Use:

Although this manual is written as a text book for those interested in certification, it is just as valuable for those of you only interested in self-healing methods.

Your Unfolding Path

Say not, "I have found the truth", but rather, "I have found a truth."
Say not, "I have found the path of the soul", but rather,
"I have met the soul walking upon my path."
For the soul walks upon all paths.
The soul walks not upon a line, neither does it grow like a reed.
The soul unfolds itself, like a lotus of countless petals.

Kahlil Gibran

GETTING CERTIFIED:

Healing Arts Practitioner and Holistic Health Consultant Certification Course

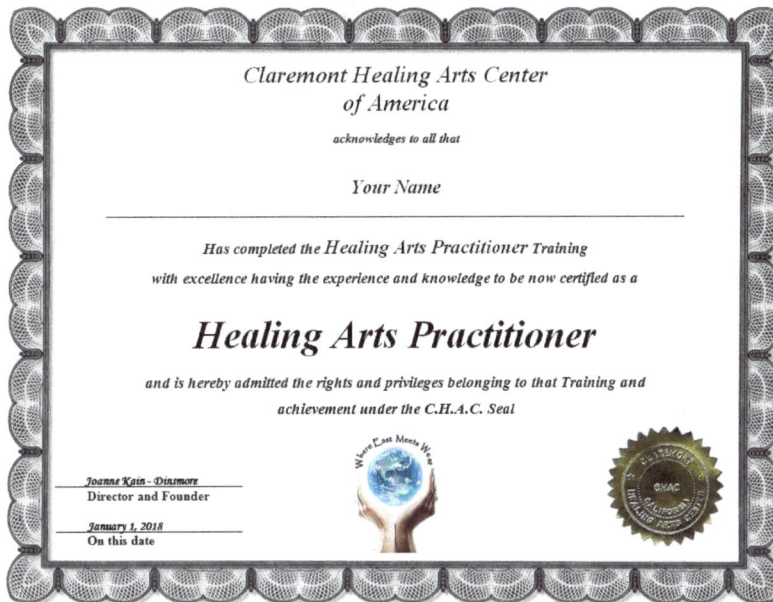

Claremont Healing Arts Center
of America

acknowledges to all that

Your Name

Has completed the *Healing Arts Practitioner* Training
with excellence having the experience and knowledge to be now certified as a

Healing Arts Practitioner

and is hereby admitted the rights and privileges belonging to that Training and achievement under the C.H.A.C. Seal

Joanne Kain - Dinsmore
Director and Founder

January 1, 2018
On this date

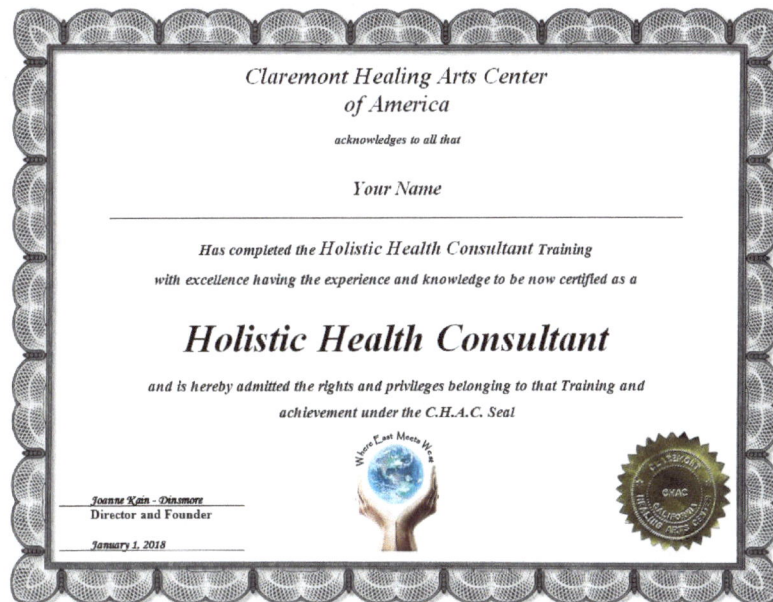

Claremont Healing Arts Center
of America

acknowledges to all that

Your Name

Has completed the *Holistic Health Consultant* Training
with excellence having the experience and knowledge to be now certified as a

Holistic Health Consultant

and is hereby admitted the rights and privileges belonging to that Training and achievement under the C.H.A.C. Seal

Joanne Kain - Dinsmore
Director and Founder

January 1, 2018

About the Claremont Healing Arts Center of America

This course is offered by the Claremont Healing Arts Center in Claremont, California. Our Center has been successful in private practice as well as training Healing Arts Practitioners since 1994.

Respected as a Holistic Health educational center, we have worked with people from all walks of life: from individual clients to organizations such as hospitals, recovery centers, senior centers and insurance health plans.

Our Mission Statement: To instruct and educate persons in the various forms of holistic and healing arts, in order that they may heal themselves and educate others, which, in turn, facilitates exponential healing of our world.

What is a Healing Arts Practitioner (HP)?

Holistic health is a growing field. At the time of this writing, a healing practitioner is someone certified by a Healing Arts Center, having completed courses in various natural healing techniques such as Reiki, reflexology, aromatherapy, Shaman Stone healing, hypnotherapy and meditation. This is just a sampling of the many techniques available today.

Licensing: Currently in America, there is no nationwide or individual state licensing for an HP and therefore no designated description of that title. This makes the individual practitioner responsible to hold a high level of integrity when practicing any healing technique on others.

Ethics: The practitioner is responsible to ensure, first and foremost, the overall well- being and safety of themselves and their clients. They are always to maintain professional boundaries. They must have an extensive knowledge of and experience in their field of healing, as well as knowing their own limitations. They need to know when to refer their client to another qualified professional, such as a counselor, therapist or medical doctor.

What is a Holistic Health Consultant (HHC)?

Holistic Health Consultants assist their clients in creating the best plan for their overall healing and wellness. This may include a referral list geared towards the health needs of the body, mind and spirit.

As an HHC, you may also offer seminars and workshops in many organizations as an educator and gain an enormous amount of fulfillment in doing so.

Licensing: HHC's may obtain a city license as a general "Holistic Health Consultant" and practice accordingly, including your Healing Arts Practitioner work.

Other legalities: Under the law, before you may touch someone in a healing arts practice, you must be either a licensed masseuse or an ordained minister. If you are not planning on becoming a licensed masseuse, then refer to the resource page at the back of this manual for the Universal Life Church website for more information on becoming ordained in your state or country. The one-time cost is nominal and allows you to legally place your hands on a client during a healing when appropriate.

Benefits of this Manual:

☐ *Self Help Tools for Body, Mind and Spirit*

☐ *A complete workbook containing all the requirements for the option of certification as a HP and HHC*

☐ *Obtaining credentials as a certified professional*

☐ *Additional credits for existing degrees (i.e. some universities will accept outside certification as elective credits)*

☐ *Materials for building your clientele*

☐ *How to establish your own business*

☐ *How and why to network with professional organizations*

☐ *Ongoing email support from the Claremont Healing Arts Center*

☐ *Becoming an educator in the field of Healing Arts and Holistic Health via workshops and seminars*

☐ *Certification / Life Skill experience for possible credits towards future state licensing if it becomes available.*

FAQ
(Frequently Asked Questions)

Can anyone be a healer?

Absolutely! It is an innate ability to be developed should you choose to do so. The vibration of compassion, in itself, is a healing emotion. The desire to develop hands-on healing skills often is elicited by that inherent guide, the inner compass for creative expression; your soul's yearning, if you will.

If you are drawn to learn something, your consciousness is longing to manifest growth towards fulfillment.

I have known so many people who wanted to do this or that and were too afraid and insecure to even try. Sadly, I watched them grow older by the year, unhappy and bitter from the stagnation and lack of fulfillment.

This is why it is so important to work through the obstacles blocking your potential to blossom and therefore gain the freedom of goals achieved. Once you stop being a participant in your inner life, you stop living.

In this manual there is a self-help section recommended for this very purpose. And since you have picked up this book, you are already willing to explore a door for expansion of your inner life.

Just like learning any new skill, it takes time to excel. Some people will be more inherently talented than others, wherein the skill becomes an art form. Regardless, everyone can benefit in learning these skills.

Is it about being psychic or a medium?

Not necessarily. However, do not be surprised if your intuition expands. There is a sizable difference between being psychic and being a medium.

A medium is a person who has access to spirits and allows the spirits to talk through him/her. A psychic is a person whose intuition is highly developed and is able to pick up vibrational information. For example, in our HP classes, we have a "psychometry" night. Each student brings an item to class from a friend (a watch, a piece of jewelry or some other trinket). We put the items in one pile. Then, each student chooses one of the items to "read" instinctually. The students will hold their chosen item and write down anything that comes to mind. (Locations, colors, names, gender, emotions, careers etc.) This is a fun exercise. And often, accuracy increases with practice.

So we all have the ability to different degrees, but it is not a requirement to become a healer.

What can I learn from this course?

As much as you want. You can learn how to heal yourself and help others and/or learn how to become a professional and start a practice of your own. The choice is yours. In either case, you will greatly benefit from the course.

Holistic Health Introduction

Understanding holistic health comes with time and through personal experiences. Every "body" is unique, so it takes a sampling of alternatives to discover what *your* body will respond to best. Some of us gain results from herbal remedies or homoeopathy while others respond better to imagery, yoga, aromatherapy etc. Understand that all natural healing modalities are a cumulative process. This means it *takes time* for the body to be nourished and trained to assimilate and respond to the natural supplement introduced. You can expect anywhere from 3 weeks to 3 months to feel results. The longer you maintain your regimen, the better the results.

This is not a quick fix but well worth your time and effort if you focus on the long term results.

Any stress to the body will create eventual breakdown and pain. Adding holistic perspective to your health regimen means adding a little TLC to the physical, emotional, mental and spiritual aspects of your being.

We are not made up of the isolated parts of a body-machine. We are many parts working as a whole, every part being interconnected. Therefore, your mental and emotional stresses will eventually affect your physical health. In turn, physical pain or discomfort may stress you mentally, which puts more stress on the physical and so on. This is the typical cycle that can cause further deterioration.

You can get off at any station along this track, thus preventing more damage and even healing to some degree the wounds you already carry.

Is this not worth your time, patience, exploration and determination?
Yes and you can do it!

Suggested Holistic Therapies

These therapies are only a few of the large number available in the Holistic Health field. Once you start with one, you will find yourself drawn into others.

- **Herbals/vitamin supplements**
- **Homeopathy**
- **Massage**
- **Acupuncture/acupressure**
- **Aromatherapy**
- **Ayurvedics**
- **Yoga, Tai Chi**
- **Journaling**

- **Imagery**
- **Energy Healing**
- **Meditation**
- **Counseling**
- **Support groups**
- **Affirmations**
- **Physical exercise**
- **Nutrition (i.e. more alkaline vs. acid foods, food combining)**

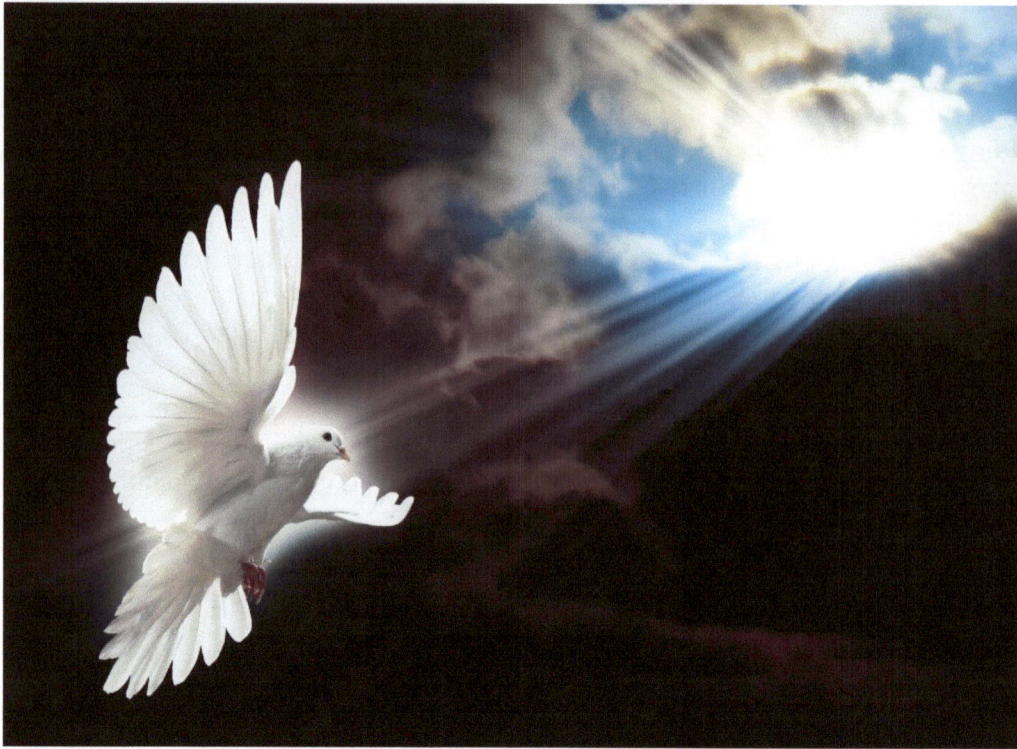

Words of Wisdom

Our deepest fear is not that we are inadequate; our deepest fear is that we are powerful beyond measure.

It is our light, not our darkness that most frightens us.

We ask ourselves who am I to be brilliant, gorgeous, talented and fabulous? You are a child of God.

You playing small does not serve the world.

There is nothing enlightened about shrinking so that other people won't feel insecure around you.

We were born to make manifest the glory of God that is everyone.

And as we let go of our own fear, our presence automatically liberates others.

Nelson Mandela, 1995

Chapter 2

Self Growth & Discovery

"You cannot know yourself without healing and you cannot heal yourself without knowing"
DOUG DINSMORE

The Tibetan Book of Living and Dying
Paths of Perception

The following poem speaks to us all. It is called "Autobiography in Five Chapters" by Sogyal Rinpoche's *The Tibetan Book of Living and Dying*.

1)   **I walk down the street.**
There is a deep hole in the sidewalk.
I fall in.
I am lost… I am hopeless.
It isn't my fault.
It takes me forever to find a way out.

2)   **I walk down the same street.**
There is a deep hole in the sidewalk.
I pretend I don't see it.
I fall in again.
I can't believe I'm in the same place.
But it isn't my fault.
It still takes a long time to get out.

3)   **I walk down the same street.**
There is a deep hole in the sidewalk.
I see it is there.
I still fall in… it's a habit.
My eyes are open.
I know where I am.
It is my fault.
I get out immediately.

4)   **I walk down the same street.**
There is a deep hole in the sidewalk.
I walk around it.

5)   **I walk down another street.**

We are Spirit-born in a human seed with the opportunity to flourish in purpose and expression.

This soulful human existence is both difficult and magnificent in experience; personal and global in significance.

Each one of us has the capability and responsibility to nurture our own development through the pursuit of self-awareness, growth and discover. There are no shortcuts to enlightenment and fulfillment. There are however, many paths to choose from in getting there.

At 15 years old, I walked down a street and this is where it took me…

Symptoms of Suppressed Anger & Fear

Sometimes we hide our anger or fear even from ourselves, (or so we think). Here are some symptoms that indicate that these issues are arising from the subconscious. They need to be addressed in order to be free to live a full and healthy life. This chapter offers several exercises to gain valuable self knowledge.

- Procrastination and depression
- Loss of interests
- Isolation and self pity
- Sarcastic humor and cynicism
- Having to be in control or perfectionism
- Demanding to be right
- Avoiding commitments
- Discomfort with stillness or silence
- Pressure to please others at any cost
- Controlled monotone speaking
- Condescension
- Feeling like you are a victim in life
- Judging others and yourself
- Envy of others' achievements
- Habitual lateness
- Nervousness with an authority figure
- Over-reacting
- Expecting the "other shoe to drop"
- Lying easily
- Addictions
- Difficulty sleeping through the night
- Clenched jaws and hunched shoulders
- Grinding the teeth during sleep

Positive Affirmations

Affirmations are not just phrases or words repeated without meaning. They are a way to change an attitude, idea, feeling or behavior. If you feel stuck in a negative thought process, affirmations can help you to release it and to manifest what you really want.

- Right now and for the rest of the day, I will respect my own boundaries and those of others without question.
- Today I will take the chance and show vulnerability with someone that I trust.
- When I am complimented today, I will hold it dear to my heart and let it feed my soul for the entire day.
- Today I will imitate a behavior I admire in someone else.
- Just for today I will let go of control and trust the unknown.
- I am a child of the Divine, precious and worthy of all that entails.
- My inner and outer beauty radiates today.
- I love myself without condition or exception.
- Today I will allow myself to rest and rejuvenate because I need it.
- I am worthy and deserving of love, serenity, peace and prosperity.
- I forgive myself and others for any hurts real or imagined.
- I forgive myself for accepting less love and respect than I honestly deserved.
- I am not alone. My spirit is connected with everyone in the universe and the Divine.
- I am willing to make different choices to change an unhealthy pattern.
- I am more giving to others today.
- Just for today, I will not worry. I know all I need is provided by the Universe.
- I am re-awakening my creativity today.
- I am fully alive and grateful for all I am and all I have received.
- This moment is good....now this moment is good.

Encourage your client to write an affirmation and read it daily for 30 days.

Introduction to the Exercises
Layers of the Onion

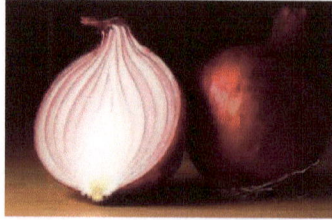

The purpose of the following exercises is to begin and continue to self-evaluate. Perhaps you have had counseling and have already worked on these issues. Please, do them anyway. No one is ever completely finished growing and self-actualizing. It is an on-going process and can be an inspiring journey.

"Progress, not perfection" is one of the 12 step program's mottos and, indeed, holds true. I've always liked the metaphor for growth as a comparison to the layers of the onion. Layer by layer we shed a skin, make a shift in awareness and go deeper towards the core of our truth. The intent is to reveal and access the core, which is the authentic and freed self.

"Authentic" self is when the inside matches the outside; you know who you are; you need not hide who you are and you honor that inner compass when making choices in life. It is not a destination however, it is an ever-learning Life Walk. As you get closest to the core, the layers seem to become more difficult to shed because they are holding onto the remaining addictive aspects of ourselves and often the toughest to release or perhaps want to let go of. We have all developed life- long defenses to cope with emotional hardships but, as we get older, these coping mechanisms do not serve us as well and it's time to put down the shields. How can you be free if you're behind the walls you built to keep others (from hurting you) out?

When Mary began counseling, her first layer she chose to address was her desire to quit smoking. She achieved that goal and felt great about herself. Quickly, behind that smoke screen she discovered the next layer of the onion: a lifetime of unresolved anger. But brave and willing, Mary walked through each issue from revelations to resolutions and felt even freer. Beneath that layer, she learned to face her fears and grieve the past. After that came development of trust and hope. The following layer involved building self worth and establishing boundaries, then working towards new goals and exploring her spirituality. While exploring this she discovered that, beneath it all, was her reliance on toxic relationships. This was a major revelation and a result of the work she had done in tearing down the walls of avoidance. After years of progress, living and learning, she came face to face with this core issue- the toughest to face and resolve because it carried the most pain to have to feel again. She spent her whole life avoiding the pain of her repressed childhood abuse. But that inner child had been running her life, by repeatedly choosing to remain in relationships with abusive men. Subconsciously, Mary was desperately seeking from men the love and approval she never had from her abusers and, of course, this would fail which would continue the cycle of her worthlessness and hopelessness, confusion and mistrust of life. Mary faced her abuse and abusers and learned how to stop her self-sabotaging choices. Overcoming a lifetime of skewed perceptions caused by emotional traumas is not an easy task.
Mary developed the courage to heal very painful issues and facing her greatest pain gave her, her greatest gift - herself.

From Mary: "I had no idea that quitting smoking would open up Pandora's Box. I had no idea I could be so strong to do this but I am so glad I did. It was like living a nightmare and not knowing why. I just thought I was fucked up and that was that. I feel like I'm alive for the first time and I like who I am now."

14

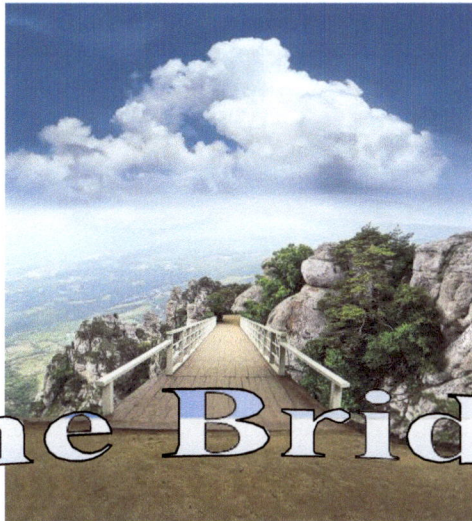

The Bridge

"I ONLY WENT OUT FOR A WALK AND FINALLY CONCLUDED TO STAY OUT TILL SUNDOWN, FOR GOING OUT, I FOUND, WAS REALLY GOING IN."

JOHN MUIR

To begin the process of self-exploration, we must start by crossing the bridges within ourselves in order to reach the other side. From there we can begin to identify what we'd like to change about ourselves and start mapping out how we will go about it.

Take a look at the process from column 1 to column 4 in exercise "Exploring the Self" on the next page. It is like walking across a bridge. You are walking from the past to the future. The walk itself takes place in the present. At first, you will be walking backwards, facing the past yet progressing towards the future. You need to, in order to recognize the origins of your inner conflicts. You need to better understand it all, to gather information and grieve the losses. Then, somewhere along the path, you will find that you have turned around, still on the bridge, but now facing the future. This is the reward for your hard work and, from that point on, it just gets better and better.

Only a person who has walked that bridge can be an ethical and effective healer. You must do you own inner work or you can do unintentional harm to a vulnerable, trusting client.

Making significant change carries three cyclic components:

1. Cognitive: how you think and what you believe.
2. Behavioral: how you act according to what you believe.
3. Emotional: how you feel as a result of your actions.

Example: Your underlying (ie: cognitive) belief is that you are an inadequate person. You will choose situations and take action to reinforce that belief (ie: behavioral) which will in turn make you feel even more of an inadequate person (ie: emotional).

I had a very funny moment with one of my clients. We were discussing his cognitive script. I asked him what his inner voice tells him about himself most often. He said, "That I'm a piece of shit."

So, we talked at length about the meaning of worthiness and agreed he would mentally re-script that voice whenever it comes up.

The following week when we met, I asked him if he had made any progress. He enthusiastically said,

"Yes, when I heard the voice tell me I was a piece of shit, I said, 'No! I am a WORTHY piece of shit!'"

15

Oh yes, we laughed and hey, it's a start. Besides, you should always be able to laugh in counseling. In fact, I believe humor is a great healing factor.

He has continued his journey and accepts his responsibility as an adult to do so. He knows he has to, for himself and others. He often and adamantly says that he needs to break the chain of insanity and dysfunction in his family patterns and lineage. What a brave man.

Healing is only as difficult as you choose it to be. Embrace the journey with hope and faith in yourself. Just walk it, one step at a time. Yes, it is all worth it. John Bradshaw, author of several self-help books, says it best, "The only way out is through." Reflect on this: What is keeping you from letting go of unhealthy people, places and things? I find that the answer is often the same: the unresolved wounds of the past.

Progress begins with cognitive re-scripting, followed by changing behavior to match the new thinking/beliefs and finally the emotional joy will reinforce the new scripts. This is the intention of this exercise.

Now, as you work through this exercise, honestly evaluate your inner child issues. Toxic emotions come from this stuck psyche. While it was not your fault that you were exposed to toxic emotions as a child, it is your responsibility now, as an adult, to heal and change the cycle.

Toxic emotions are an immaturity, no different than an undeveloped, weakened tree. It just hasn't been nourished enough to grow and blossom. Immaturity is not a shameful state. All it means is undeveloped. At what age are you stuck...5,12,16? Knowing this is an important part achieving your goal. Your goal is to become a healthy adult, capable of mature love and mature self-respect.

Exploring the Self

Exercise

Every emotion is important, needed and valid. However, every emotion has two faces, like a coin. For example, there is healthy anger and unhealthy anger. Anger is appropriate for setting boundaries. Fear is appropriate as an alarm system. Unhealthy emotions are toxic, unproductive and can eat you alive. You can begin to recognize when an emotion becomes toxic: you can't let it go: you feel like a victim most of the time and you become an over-reactive person.

In this first exercise, you will see a list of emotions, each with a brief description. Feel free to *add to the descriptions in order to personalize them as you reflect on your own history.* Do the same for each column.

- The "**Opposite**" column suggests some goals.
- The "**Solution**" column suggests the action or method to reach the goal.
- The "**Affirmation**" column re-scripts your thinking and underlying beliefs.

To make significant changes, truly life-altering changes, can take blood, sweat, tears and downright grit to accomplish. Never give up. Always persevere. I have seen hundreds of clients transform but only those who persevered. It still amazes me when I hear from a client I worked with 15 years ago, wanting to thank me again because they are happy and productive. I tell them all the same thing, "All I did was give you the tools. You're the one who did the work."

Exploring the Self: Emotions and their Properties

Emotion	*Description*	*Opposite*	*Soul-ution*	*Affirmation*
Anger	Wanting to hurt back, or control others to protect from being hurt.	Acceptance, calm, understanding.	Compassion, personal therapeutic emotional growth. Forgiveness of others. An understanding of their history.	*I understand and accept that all humans struggle on this life path. I can only help myself to help make the world a better place. I can forgive.*
Gluttony	I want "*more*" Consumption to excess: Food, drugs, thrill seeking, attention, addiction to emotions.	Self discipline.	Self respect, patience, holding off instant gratification (impulsiveness).	*I release my need to fill my emptiness with external sources. I am filled with the guidance of God's Love and Self Love. I have the power to choose.*
Jealousy	I should have that and you shouldn't.	Generosity.	Gratitude for all you currently have. Achieving goals for what you want. Self acceptance for your limitations.	*I honor my abilities and limitations. I research whatever I want to achieve. I celebrate what others have achieved.*
Sloth	Laziness -I don't feel like doing even though I could. Fear, perfectionism.	Enthusiasm, purpose, flexibility.	Taking initiative, achieving small goals one at a time, planning ahead.	*I feel so good as I've finished this task. I release the need to be perfect. I enjoy the process, step by step.*

Emotion	Description	Opposite	Soul-ution	Affirmation
Lust	Excessive sexual desire, fame, glory, egocentric.	Satisfaction.	Personal morals, self control, regard for others.	*I respect myself and others. I fully appreciate all that I have . I take nothing for granted now. My fulfillment comes from within.*
Greed	Unwillingness to share money, time, material things, hoarding.	Philanthropy, willingness to share.	Small acts of kindness, selflessness.	*I find that giving to others is freeing. All the Love given and received fulfills me. I am filled with self respect.*
Pride	Superiority, arrogance; comparing yourself to others. Fear of being humiliated.	Humility.	Honest self analysis, desire to learn from others.	*As an adult I know there are those who know more than me and know less than me. I am humble and wise to learn from others and grateful for the help of others.*
No Pride	Self beratement, low self worth.	Confidence.	Distinguishing between humility and humiliation. Allowing healthy pride/confidence for a job well done or healthy choice made.	*As an adult, I release the need to listen to my past. I am proud for all I have achieved. I am allowed to feel confident.*
Fear	Helplessness, having no control, anticipating the worst. Immobilization or rushing for distraction.	Confidence, ability, faith, calm.	Initiative / doing, collect information, open to grow, interpersonal communication, meditation.	*I am able to collect the information I need to make choices and have options. I am worthy of asking for guidance. Everything will work out with action. I am safe and capable.*
Neediness	Insatiable; an aspect of gluttony.	Self trust, emotionally self reliant.	Parent myself. Seeking help from counselor. Inner Child work.	*I can reflect on my own emotional issues. I understand this is my wounded child. My adult self makes choices. I like being an adult.*
Shame	Unworthiness, inferiority.	Healthy pride, self acceptance.	Objective feedback. Honest self analysis. Forgiveness of self and others. Acknowledgement of positive acts. Inner Child work.	*I am brave enough to review my life with others who are trustworthy . I am able to accept the truth and make amends where I can. I forgive myself and others. I have grown by all I've learned, I see the good I've done. I can live in the present now.*
Sad	Hopelessness. Loss of something of value.	Contentment, serenity, joy. State of grace.	Appreciation, gratitude, interpersonal communication, seeking faith and purpose, taking action, perseverance. Helping others.	*I actively seek help and understanding of my True purpose in life. I am not alone. I have depth and sensitivity and my path is special. I can touch the world with my God given gifts.*
Love	Compassion, affection, tenderness, giving, receiving, strong.	Apathy, arrogant, callous, taking, weak.	Forgive others that treat you disrespectfully, put yourself in their shoes, be open and honest, be positive.	*I am compassionate. I give and receive love with every breath I take. I show love to myself and all those around me. The more I love, the happier I am.*

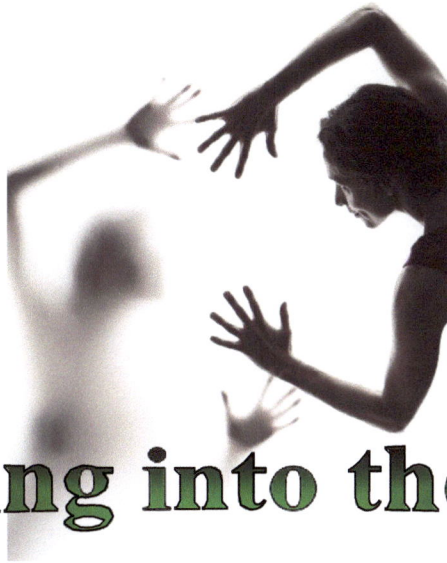

Delving into the Self

Exercise

"IN THE MIDST OF WINTER, I FOUND WITHIN ME AN INVINCIBLE SUMMER."
Albert Camus

Now we get into the nitty gritty. This exercise should be worked on patiently and methodically. Don't cheat yourself of revelations by racing through it. Write all your answers in <u>a separate notebook so you can keep these blank pages for clients</u>. For clients, this will be an awakening or a reminder of therapeutic issues they may need to address. As a healer and holistic health consultant, you are helping them become aware of the emotional or mental issues that may be affecting their physical and energetic imbalances. You are only awakening and balancing the energy systems of the body, mind, emotions and spirit while encouraging strength and ability to seek growth, to become a more whole and centered individual.

You know now that you must do this work before you can guide anyone else. You are in a position of helping them to help themselves and they are counting on you to be capable of doing so. Be honest with them and refer them to professionals when you recognize your limitations in serving them.

<u>In this exercise, answer each question as best you can and write as much as you want to in your notebook. Notice that there is a 30-day affirmations commitment at the end.</u> You will find, after you have completed the entire exercise, that your affirmations have a common thread. Create the affirmation, (sentence or paragraph) that clearly states your new belief. This affirmation then becomes your 30-day written statement. You will be amazed how many habits you can change with this kind of reinforcing practice.

An affirmation has to be believable to your core self. You cannot state, for example, "I am rich", if your deepest belief is "No, I don't really believe that." So, when creating an affirmation, use only words you can accept as true for who you are right now. "I am rich" can become "I am willing to receive more." An affirmation is not a wish. It is a realistic re-framing of your thoughts, one progressive step and statement at a time. And remember, a thought change must be followed by a behavior change. To receive more, you need to give more and the thought behind that behavior would be "I lovingly give to others as I continue to prosper."

Now, let's start the exercise. Notice, I begin with the Serenity Prayer. This is my favorite quote. I live by it. It is framed and hung in my bathroom at home as a daily reminder. It reminds me to think and act as a maturing person. It is a very powerful tool for me. You will see that I have expanded on each phrase and I encourage you to do the same. Make it your own and let this be a guide as you reflect on each question to be answered.

The first page deals with the first emotion of anger. Here, you will see examples of answers for each question. There will, no doubt, be more than one anger scenario you will want to address. You may want to list each event first and then follow the questionnaire for each one. Don't be surprised if, by the end of this exercise, you have 20 or more completed pages. Indulge yourself. Be patient. Enjoy the freedom of letting it all out and releasing it. This is your opportunity to allow yourself to express your feelings while exercising hope and change. Every step in the walk of life is a choice in attitude as to where you end up. It may not always be easy at first, but in the end, it's always worth the trek. Another motto from the 12-step program is, "It works if you work it; it won't if you don't."

God, grant me the serenity
to accept the things I cannot change;
courage to change the things I can and
wisdom to know the difference.
Reinhold Niebuhr

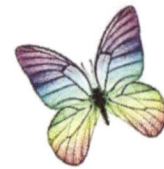

What it means:

"to accept the things I cannot change": *You can only learn from it.* To force change is to lose the lesson being taught by the experience.

"courage to change the things I can": *Yourself* is the only thing you can change, the only thing you have power over. You have *choices*, which may allow change.

"wisdom to know the difference": Includes a *new way of thinking.* Having gone through the lesson, you have experienced it and gained wisdom from it, therefore seeing the difference between choices.

Within the next few pages we will begin to explore the foundations of some of the more common emotional states all people experience. Follow the directions on the first page and continue for the subsequent pages and you will begin to receive a greater understanding of who you are presently.

From this exercise, you will have the choice to "change the things you can" and understand more of the "wisdom to know the difference".

Delving into the Self
Example

Fill in the blanks and become aware of your true self. The more honest you are with your*self,* the more your *Self* will be honest with you!

1. Anger (*fury, rage, irritation*)

A.) I get angry when I

I don't stand up for myself and say "no". Or don't remove myself from situations that do not serve my emotional/spiritual growth.

B.) This anger reminds me of (how does this anger relate to your past?)

My failed marriage. All the times I "should" have said no or stopped some behavior. I didn't do it! ARRGGHH!! Taking more time for others than for myself. Not leaving toxic jobs or *obviously* unhealthy relationships.

C.) This is how it has affected my life as an adult

I find myself in situations I really don't want to be in any longer or I stay in relationships that aren't working for fear of confrontation about the issue at hand or fear of being alone.

D.) My Inner Child script says

"They won't listen to me anyway! Don't even try! My voice, idea, opinion means nothing! It's *worthless, stupid!* Better to stay quiet, just go along with it, even if I don't like it or know it's wrong. It'll get better *later."* The adult knows intellectually that "later" never comes, the resentment and frustration builds instead and adds another layer of crap to the dumping ground of my self worth, my self esteem.

E.) What I choose to change is

My perspective. Every time that dialogue comes up I will not ignore it but observe it, make note of it and move ahead by giving my opinion, idea, suggestion anyway, regardless of the fear. Tell my inner child she is safe and worthy.

F.) I am willing to replace the feeling of victimhood by writing this affirmation 30 days without exception

My opinions and ideas are just as worthy as anyone else's. If I feel I need to remove myself from a situation because I believe it to be wrong or its time for me to move on I will say so. I will confront with compassion. I will nurture my inner child to let her voice be heard. I *am* worthy!

Notes: _____

_____

Delving into the Self

An Exercise for Self-Discovery & Transformation

Fill in the blanks and become aware of your true self. The more honest you are with yourself the more yourself will be honest with you.

1. Anger (*fury, rage, irritation*)

A.) I get angry when _____

_____

_____

B.) This anger reminds me of (how does this anger relate to your past?) _____

_____

_____

C.) This is how it has affected my life as an adult _____

_____

_____

D.) My Inner Child script says _____

_____

_____

E.) What I choose to change is _____

_____

_____

F.) I am willing to replace the feeling of victimhood by writing this affirmation 30 days without exception

_____

_____

_____

Notes: _____

_____

_____

_____

2. Gluttony (*excess*)

A.) I practice gluttony when _____

_____

_____

B.) This gluttony reminds me of (how does this gluttony relate to your past?) _____

_____

_____

C.) This is how it has affected my life as an adult _____

_____

_____

D.) My Inner Child script says _____

_____

_____

E.) What I choose to change is _____

_____

_____

F.) I am willing to replace the feeling of victimhood by writing this affirmation 30 days without exception

_____

_____

_____

Notes: _____

_____

_____

_____

_____

_____

_____

_____

_____

_____

3. Jealousy (*envy, suspicion, distrust*)

A.) I get jealous when _____

_____

_____

B.) This jealousy reminds me of (how does this jealousy relate to your past?) _____

_____

_____

C.) This is how it has affected my life as an adult _____

_____

_____

D.) My Inner Child script says _____

_____

_____

E.) What I choose to change is _____

_____

_____

F.) I am willing to replace the feeling of victimhood by writing this affirmation 30 days without exception

_____

_____

_____

Notes: _____

_____

_____

_____

_____

_____

_____

_____

_____

_____

4. Sloth (*laziness, idleness, inactivity, apathy*)

A.) I get idle when _____

_____

_____

B.) This idleness reminds me of (how does this idleness relate to your past?) _____

_____

_____

_____

C.) This is how it has affected my life as an adult _____

_____

_____

D.) My Inner Child script says _____

_____

_____

E.) What I choose to change is _____

_____

_____

F.) I am willing to replace the feeling of victimhood by writing this affirmation 30 days without exception

_____

_____

_____

Notes: _____

_____

_____

_____

_____

_____

_____

_____

_____

5. Lust (*yearn, desire, envy*)

A.) I get lustful when _____

_____

_____

B.) This lust reminds me of (how does this lust relate to your past?) _____

_____

_____

C.) This is how it has affected my life as an adult _____

_____

_____

D.) My Inner Child script says _____

_____

_____

E.) What I choose to change is _____

_____

_____

F.) I am willing to replace the feeling of victimhood by writing this affirmation 30 days without exception

_____

_____

_____

Notes: _____

_____

_____

_____

_____

_____

_____

_____

_____

_____

6. Greed (*self indulgence, insatiability*)

A.) I get greedy when _____

_____

_____

B.) This greed reminds me of (how does this greed relate to your past?) _____

_____

_____

C.) This is how it has affected my life as an adult _____

_____

_____

D.) My Inner Child script says _____

_____

_____

E.) What I choose to change is _____

_____

_____

F.) I am willing to replace the feeling of victimhood by writing this affirmation 30 days without exception

_____

_____

_____

Notes: _____

_____

_____

_____

_____

_____

_____

_____

_____

7A. Pride (*self importance*)

A.) I get prideful when _____

_____

_____

B.) This pride reminds me of (how does this pride relate to your past?) _____

_____

_____

C.) This is how it has affected my life as an adult _____

_____

_____

D.) My Inner Child script says _____

_____

_____

E.) What I choose to change is _____

_____

_____

F.) I am willing to replace the feeling of victimhood by writing this affirmation 30 days without exception

_____

_____

_____

Notes: _____

_____

_____

_____

_____

_____

_____

_____

_____

_____

7 B. No Pride (*lack of self importance, low self worth*)

A.) I feel worthless when _____

_____

_____

B.) This lack of pride reminds me of (how does this worthless feeling relate to your past?)

_____

_____

_____

C.) This is how it has affected my life as an adult _____

_____

_____

D.) My Inner Child script says _____

_____

_____

E.) What I choose to change is _____

_____

_____

F.) I am willing to replace the feeling of victimhood by writing this affirmation 30 days without exception

_____

_____

_____

Notes: _____

_____

_____

_____

_____

_____

_____

_____

8. Fear (*anxiety, worry, dread*)

A.) I get fearful when _____

_____

_____

B.) This fearfulness reminds me of (how does this Fear relate to your past?) _____

_____

_____

C.) This is how it has affected my life as an adult _____

_____

_____

D.) My Inner Child script says _____

_____

_____

E.) What I choose to change is _____

_____

_____

F.) I am willing to replace the feeling of victimhood by writing this affirmation 30 days without exception

_____

_____

_____

Notes: _____

_____

_____

_____

_____

_____

_____

_____

_____

9. Neediness (*want, hardship, destitution*)

A.) I get needy when _____

_____

_____

B.) This neediness reminds me of (how does this neediness relate to your past?)_____

_____

_____

C.) This is how it has affected my life as an adult _____

_____

_____

D.) My Inner Child script says _____

_____

_____

E.) What I choose to change is _____

_____

_____

F.) I am willing to replace the feeling of victimhood by writing this affirmation 30 days without exception

_____

_____

_____

Notes:_____

_____

_____

_____

_____

_____

_____

_____

_____

10. Shame (*disgrace, embarrassment, dishonor*)

A.) I get shameful when _____

_____

_____

B.) This shame reminds me of (how does this shame relate to your past?) _____

_____

_____

C.) This is how it has affected my life as an adult _____

_____

_____

D.) My Inner Child script says _____

_____

_____

E.) What I choose to change is _____

_____

_____

F.) I am willing to replace the feeling of victimhood by writing this affirmation 30 days without exception

_____

_____

_____

Notes: _____

_____

_____

_____

_____

_____

_____

_____

_____

11. Sad (*depressed, miserable, gloomy*)

A.) I get sad when _____

_____

_____

B.) This sadness reminds me of (how does this sadness relate to your past?) _____

_____

_____

C.) This is how it has affected my life as an adult _____

_____

_____

D.) My Inner Child script says _____

_____

_____

E.) What I choose to change is _____

_____

_____

F.) I am willing to replace the feeling of victimhood by writing this affirmation 30 days without exception

_____

_____

_____

Notes: _____

_____

_____

_____

_____

_____

_____

_____

_____

12. Love (*affection, tenderness, devotion*)

A.) I feel loved when _____

_____

_____

B.) This reminds me of (how does this relate to your past?) _____

_____

_____

C.) This is how it has affects my life as an adult _____

_____

_____

D.) My Inner Child script says _____

_____

_____

E.) What I choose to change is _____

_____

_____

F.) I am willing to replace the feeling of victimhood by writing this affirmation 30 days without exception

_____

_____

_____

Notes: _____

_____

_____

_____

_____

_____

_____

_____

_____

Tending your Inner Garden- Imagery

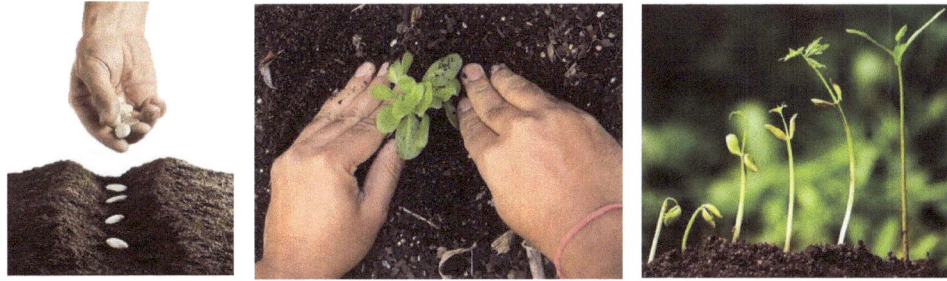

Our inner selves can be likened to a garden. The garden is first filled with fertile soil to ensure the rooting of a seed. Water and sunlight nourishes its growth for fruition and harvest - the goal intended and achieved. But even in a thriving garden there are weeds. Periodically, we need to clear out those weeds that can strangle or starve a plant from growing, reaching maturity and fruition.

In this imagery the weeds will represent the negative thoughts, feelings and actions that creep into our habits and psyches. The flora, plants and blossoms will represent the manifestation of our goals and aspirations. Revisiting this imagery can often produce fascinating and profound shifts in attitude resulting in actual positive change. Perhaps this is due to the use of the creative mind rather than solely using the left brain linear process in re-scripting patterns of thought. I still visit this place of clarity a few times a year and see the underlying truth within myself.

I suggest you revisit this imagery every two weeks at first.

Imagery

Sit comfortably and take in several slow deep breaths. Allow a warmth of relaxation to envelope your entire body like a soft sun-lit cloud descending upon you. Let this relaxation flow into your skin, muscles, organs and bones. As you breathe, relax even deeper now… worries and stresses just melt away. A waterfall of deep relaxation washes over you and within you. You are free and your lungs are free, open and relaxed. Breathe and sink in deeper and deeper… (pause)

Imagine now that you are walking on a path in nature. The sunshine is healing. The blue sky is clear and the aromas of nature are fresh and cleansing. Breathe.

You now come upon a lovely fertile garden. This is your place of peace and power. All you plant here will flourish with ease. This is an empowering and positive place to visit.

You now see the first patch of weeds. These are the weeds of anger and you pull them all out by the roots and hand them to your angel, guide, or back to the universe. Take all the time you need… there is no right way or wrong way to do this. Do this now…(pause)

Now, find all the weeds of fear and pull them all out. Take your time. (pause)

Now continue pulling weeds of shame and inadequacy…(pause)

Lastly, pull out all the weeds of sadness, releasing it all…(pause)

You now have a lovely clean garden space to work with. You can now sprinkle it with rich fertilized soil. Do this now. …(pause)

Stand back. Look at your garden and the surrounding area, this beautiful fresh aromatic place. Breathe in the scents.

Now is the time to plant your seeds. Plant a seed for every goal. Plant a seed of wisdom…now of acceptance and love…now of prosperity…now of confidence…

And now plant anymore seeds you want for maturity and achievement.

Take all the time you want…When you're ready, water your garden…

Closing:
It is time to walk back to the path now. Breathe in deeply as you walk back into the room. You are now awake and refreshed as you open your eyes… The next time you visit your garden you will see surprising growth and change. Continue to weed and water with every visit.

Self-evaluation
Exercise

Here is where we begin to weed our inner garden. If you happen to have the proverbial black thumb in the physical world, be assured that in the Spirit or inner world, your thumb can be as green as the lushest forest. Answer each question for the topic listed. See the example below:

Example:
(Topic) **<u>Drinking/Drugs</u>**

1.   Where am I now? (Observation: Weed or Flower?)
I'm an overgrown weed! I tend to drink when I get really stressed or can't sleep. I'm so tired all the time and I wake up with headaches. I feel like crap most of the time.

2.   Where do I want to be? (Goal: Seed)?
Not so dependent on it. Find a healthier way to de-stress and have more energy to be happier.

3.   How can I get there? (Footwork: Water/nourish)
I gotta admit I'm addicted. Accept that it's okay to get help. I don't want to go to AA yet, but I will go talk to a counselor and learn some stress-reduction techniques. And if that doesn't work, I will go to AA.

Now it's your turn. You may want to share this with friends and family if they're receptive, but ultimately this tool is to help you realize *where you are now*, where you *want to be* and *how to get there.* Use the "Tending Your Inner Garden" meditation before and after this exercise. The answers will change with time. If you need to, use a separate notebook or journal to record your answers. Remember that being less than honest with your answers is being less than honest with *yourself.*

Self evaluation

Drinking/Drugs

1.   **Where am I now?**

_____

_____

_____

2.   **Where do I want to be?**

_____

_____

_____

3.   **How can I get there?**

_____

_____

_____

Emotional Maturity

1.   **Where am I now?**

_____

_____

_____

2.   **Where do I want to be?**

_____

_____

_____

3.   **How can I get there?**

_____

_____

_____

Self evaluation

Spiritual Life

1. **Where am I now?**

    _____

    _____

    _____

2. **Where do I want to be?**

    _____

    _____

    _____

3. **How can I get there?**

    _____

    _____

    _____

Self Worth

1. **Where am I now?**

    _____

    _____

    _____

2. **Where do I want to be?**

    _____

    _____

    _____

3. **How can I get there?**

    _____

    _____

    _____

Self evaluation

Family Life

1. Where am I now?

   _____

   _____

   _____

2. Where do I want to be?

   _____

   _____

   _____

3. How can I get there?

   _____

   _____

   _____

Personal Relationships

1. Where am I now?

   _____

   _____

   _____

2. Where do I want to be

   _____

   _____

   _____

3. How can I get there?

   _____

   _____

   _____

Self evaluation

Recreation & Hobbies

1.   **Where am I now?**

_____

_____

_____

2.   **Where do I want to be?**

_____

_____

_____

3.   **How can I get there?**

_____

_____

_____

Community

1.   **Where am I now?**

_____

_____

_____

2.   **Where do I want to be?**

_____

_____

_____

3.   **How can I get there?**

_____

_____

_____

Self evaluation

Physical Health & Fitness

1. **Where am I now?**

   _____

   _____

   _____

2. **Where do I want to be?**

   _____

   _____

   _____

3. **How can I get there?**

   _____

   _____

   _____

Sexual Health

1. **Where am I now?**

   _____

   _____

   _____

2. **Where do I want to be?**

   _____

   _____

   _____

3. **How can I get there?**

   _____

   _____

   _____

Self evaluation

Physical Home (roof over your head)

1.   **Where am I now?**

_____

_____

_____

2.   **Where do I want to be?**

_____

_____

_____

3.   **How can I get there?**

_____

_____

_____

Job

1.   **Where am I now?**

_____

_____

_____

2.   **Where do I want to be?**

_____

_____

_____

3.   **How can I get there?**

_____

_____

_____

Self evaluation

<u>Education</u>

1. **Where am I now?**

   _____

   _____

   _____

2. **Where do I want to be?**

   _____

   _____

   _____

3. **How can I get there?**

   _____

   _____

   _____

<u>Dreams/Goals</u>

1. **Where am I now?**

   _____

   _____

   _____

2. **Where do I want to be?**

   _____

   _____

   _____

3. **How can I get there?**

   _____

   _____

   _____

Do I Have a Purpose in this Life?

I am only a carpenter.
If it wasn't for you I wouldn't have a house.
I am only a trash man.
If it wasn't for you, we would be infested with toxins.
I am only a cook.
If it wasn't for you, we could never eat a fine meal.

I never finished my Masters' Degree.
I'm only teaching in elementary school.
I am a construction worker but could've been an engineer.
I wish I could've reached my potential.

These are the words I have heard from so many people I have known, including myself. I could write an entire book just on this topic of unrealized potential. Remember the Serenity Prayer?

Accept the things I cannot change.
(The dreams that didn't come to pass)
Change the things I can.
(The dreams yet to come)
And the wisdom to know the difference.

"Why, why, why didn't I get to do what I *could've* done, been what I *could've* been?" Your *potential* is not necessarily your *purpose* in this life's walk. Yet, your *true purpose* might be your gift to the world and more fulfilling than you ever imagined.

I have known very few people who knew early in life what they wanted to be and had then attained it. Yes, a small percentage (very small) have done so. The rest of us have struggled to find out; others, still unfulfilled, quit trying.

I had struggled long and hard in this life but had circumstances and obstacles not prevented me from doing what I *thought* I wanted to do, I would not have travelled on the path of spiritual richness I have obtained so far.

I started out judgmental.
Now I am compassionate.
I started out beaten.
Now I am healed.
Now that I am healed, I seek to heal others.

All of us have had dreams that didn't come to pass. But the greatest qualities within us were developed by facing life's unexpected and sometimes brutal lessons. There is only one reason we all made it through such difficult experiences: We didn't give up! You have a purpose in this life. No matter what you are doing, it matters. *You matter.*

Do not give up. Do not stop seeking your purpose and do not stop doing what it takes to make it happen, no matter how old you are, no matter what others say, no matter what obstacles seem to be in your way.

When I finished college, an 81-year-old female classmate of mine did as well. She never abandoned her dream to obtain a college degree.

How do I move forward?

We need to understand that immaturity leads to expecting instant gratification as well as fostering laziness, denial and excuses. With a lack of maturity, we fail to understand that the fears we have are simply shadows. The capacity for and the potential of maturity means that we turn on the lights and watch those shadows fade. Maybe the greatest gift we have is the potential to overcome fears and suffering.

Accept the circumstances that have altered the course in your life. Accept the choices you have made in your life and choose today to work towards another goal. It is never too late.

Cindy's obstacle and victory

"I never had to financially provide for myself until I was divorced and terrified. But I made it. I did it. I didn't like it, but I did it. I feel proud and strong and have grown so much."

Cindy didn't know she had it in her. She could have chosen to stay depressed and bitter, but chose instead to open her horizons. The job where she is working isn't her dream but she accepts that. She has started taking classes in oil painting and it is fulfilling for her. Her goal is to teach a beginner's painting class at a senior center as her hobby. She is 56 years old and has *chosen to expand herself*, something she never thought she could do, being rather shy. She feels a purpose in life, a creative unrealized expression of herself, beyond being a mother. She is a *participant* in her life walk, instead of just watching life walk by. She is overcoming her fears and doubts. Being courageous means that you're afraid, but you do it regardless of that fear, whatever "it" may be.

Julie's forced life makeover

"In the fall of 1995, after nine years of marriage, my husband and I split up. At the time, we were living in South Carolina and, after the break up, he decided to move to another state. Just a few weeks before that I had lost my car (it stopped running). Since we lived about 30 miles away from my job (or any other job for that matter), I lost that too. So there I was: no job, no car, a daughter to take care of and a house payment to make. What the heck was the *purpose* in this?

I met my husband when I was 15 and we were married about four years later. So I had never known a life without him in it. When he left, I was an empty shell. Luckily, I had friends who helped me get back in touch with my family back in California. With a duffle bag over my shoulder, the clothes on my back and my daughter in tow, we took a Greyhound bus back home. I was now relying on the kindness of family to help me through this. I had no idea of *what* to do, much less *how* to do it. Thankfully, I have really awesome family and friends. They helped me to find the path; however, *I* was the one who had to take the steps.

I knew I had hard choices to make and I made them. I went on welfare and started to put my life back together. By 1996, I had gone back to adult school to get my high school diploma. Then I started college. In 1999 I graduated from college, moved out of my mother's house, took Joanne's Healing Practioner courses (yes, the ones in this book!) and worked my way off of welfare. Sound good so far? It gets *even better*. When you first make the choice, it's like a snowball on top of a 5 mile high mountain. It gains speed and momentum and overcomes most, if not all, obstacles. By 2005, I had my first vacation by myself; I went to Oregon.

In 2007, I went on a Vision Quest, also in Oregon (see Volume 2 from the <u>Pathways to the Healing Arts</u> series). In 2008, another trip to Oregon. By this time, the snowball was *huge!* Between 2009 and 2011, I traveled to Ireland to study Celtic shamanism. Finally, also in 2011, I agreed to work with Joanne, authoring Volume 2 in the healing series, including all I've learned and experienced thus far. See? Snowball.

From those humble beginnings, I had no idea what my purpose was or would be. I simply put one foot in front of the other. In hindsight, I sometimes wonder what would have happened had my ex-husband and I stayed together. I can't imagine. So, for his contribution to this "forced life makeover", I owe him thanks. I never could have done it without that first choice."

Whether you are a teacher, a construction worker, a fast food worker, a trash man or a salesman, if you still feel unfulfilled, do what it takes to add that unrealized gift and joy to your life. Meanwhile, be proud of the valuable purpose you serve in the lives of others.

Do you have a purpose?
No matter where you are right now in this life, you are in your purpose. Waking up in the morning and taking that first step will lead you down the path where you may choose to participate in this life walk.

Now keep going!

All of these exercises are just the tip of the iceberg towards self-awareness. I hope that they've stirred you out of your complacency and sparked some curiosity. I begin every day with a blank slate, on which we start to write anew. I want you to challenge yourself to reach for more, to take advantage of all the possibilities life offers up every day and to know what it's like to feel the joy of having significance.

Keep growing!

How to be Happy
Do what it takes and then do it again!

Don't worry, be *happy*! Worry less and choose the positive. Happiness is a transient state. You will tend to be happier, both with yourself and with others when you regularly practice exercises like these.

♥ List 10 things you like about yourself. (Don't be shy, this is for your eyes only)

1) _____

_____

2) _____

_____

3) _____

_____

4) _____

_____

5) _____

_____

6) _____

_____

7) _____

_____

8) _____

_____

9) _____

_____

10) _____

_____

☺   List 5 things you don't like about yourself. (Be brave, you're making changes to **h**appy.)

1.) _____

2.) _____

3.) _____

4.) _____

5.) _____

✍   List 5 things you can choose to do to like yourself more.

1.) _____
_____

2.) _____
_____

3.) _____
_____

4.) _____
_____

5.) _____
_____

Let's go deeper

👪 Imagine that the members of your family and all the significant relationships you've had in this life were the result of your soul's choice. What lessons for growth have you had to learn? To provide for yourself? To be emotionally independent? To learn patience, compassion? To learn to compromise or to set boundaries? Maybe they just helped you to make better choices. Perhaps they taught you what you didn't want in a relationship. We are all each other's teachers. This is their gift to you (and yours to them). If you can accept the lessons and be grateful for them, you have achieved a level of enlightenment and you will be a happier person because of it.

■ List the positive things you gained from your most significant relationships.

_____
_____
_____
_____
_____
_____
_____
_____
_____
_____
_____
_____

☞ Now list 1 thing you will treat yourself to this week.

_____
_____
_____
_____

List 1 person and 1 organization you will contribute to this month. Pick one you usually wouldn't consider. Here are some examples:

♥　　Send a nice card to someone who hasn't heard from you in a while.

♥　　Donate money or time for a good cause.

♥　　Make something to donate to a Senior Center.

♥　　Volunteer for a soup kitchen.

♥　　Buy a toy for a child.

♥　　Bake cookies for someone.

♥　　Give up a prime parking spot to the other car waiting for a space.

♥　　Remember to do these things with a feeling of gratitude and unconditional love.

How to deal with the hard times

As Les Brown, my favorite motivational speaker and radio talk show host, says,

- ✓ **"When life knocks you down, try to land on your back, because as long as you can *look* up, you can *get* up."**

- ✓ **"Don't let others bring you down."**

- ✓ **"To be successful, you have to do what other people are not willing to do."**

- ✓ **"When you hear yourself thinking or saying something negative, stop and say "Cancel! Clear!" and start over."**

- ✓ **"No matter how bad it is, or how bad it gets, I am going to make it."**

A final note on happiness

One of the reasons I respect Les Brown is because he didn't have it easy in this life. From being abandoned at birth to living in poverty, he has risen above it all. But he has not forgotten the lessons from hardships. Those lessons kept him motivated to reach for more, for happiness.

Many of us have been faced with hardships. When *I* have one to face, I think of Les. If he can get up, then *I* can get up. And so can *you.*

Les says, "You have something special in you. You have greatness within you".

It's easy to be happy when everything's going your way. But it's the tough times that bring you opportunities for maturity, achievement and gained wisdom. Stay positive. That is the only way to have true happiness which is ultimately, contentment.

Now, nurture your spark and find your greatness!

The 30 Day Journal

It takes 30 days to change a pattern. I have used this simple exercise for decades and it works. You will experience a shift in your attitude, perspective and behavior. It's just like joining a gym and working out for 30 days. You feel undeniably great!

Then you start to slack off and the old unhealthy habits kick back in. If you choose to return to the gym, you reap the rewards again and if you choose to do so sooner than later you will find that exercising can become a new habit. Repetition will eventually change a pattern.

So for the next 30 days, practice these steps:

Day 1- Write in your journal everything from the past to the present that upsets or affects you. Let yourself bitch, complain or mourn. Then re-visit the Serenity Prayer and make the decision to go forward by committing to this 30 day exercise.

Day 2-30:

1. Every single time you hear yourself say a negative, sarcastic, cynical or complaining remark, immediately catch it and say: *"Cancel! Clear!"* and start your day over again.

2. Every morning, you have another chance to live in a better way.
   Say to yourself every morning for 30 days:

   "I will be a mature adult today."

   "I will re-adjust my attitude today."

   "I will be grateful today."

(You can print it out and put it on your bathroom mirror, near the coffee pot or in the car. Just make it accessible).

3. At the end of each day, answer these three questions in your journal:

   "What was I grateful for today?" (as simple as noticing a rainbow)

   "What was I proud of today?" (accomplishment)

   "What did I like about myself today?" (personality, physical appearance and interactions)

Self Esteem Exercise

Self-esteem is very important to a healthy, well-balanced life. It is not vanity or overconfidence. Rather, it is an honest view of ones' qualities as an individual. Our self-esteem suffers when we experience negativity from ourselves or others. This exercise will help remind you that we are all worthy, important, cherished and loved.

1. List 5 or more people you love:

_____   _____

_____   _____

_____   _____

_____   _____

_____   _____

2. List 5 or more people you admire and why: Names:

Why?

_____   _____

_____   _____

_____   _____

_____   _____

_____   _____

_____   _____

_____   _____

_____   _____

3. List 5 people who respect and love you:

_____

_____

_____

_____

_____

4. List 5 or more things you are grateful for:

_____

_____

_____

_____

_____

List 5 or more things you are interested in and have a knack for:

_____   _____

_____   _____

_____   _____

_____   _____

_____   _____

5.   **List 5 or more characteristics you generally like about yourself:**

_____   _____

_____   _____

_____   _____

_____   _____

_____   _____

6.   **List 5 or more characteristics you want to cultivate and nurture within yourself:**

_____   _____

_____   _____

_____   _____

_____   _____

_____   _____

_____   _____

_____   _____

_____   _____

_____   _____

7.   **List 5 or more achievements you've made in your life so far:**

_____   _____

_____   _____

_____   _____

_____   _____

_____   _____

8. **List 5 or more physical characteristics you like about yourself:**

_____   _____

_____   _____

_____   _____

_____   _____

_____   _____

9. **List 5 or more random acts of kindness you have performed for yourself, others, or the environment in your life so far:**

_____   _____

_____   _____

_____   _____

_____   _____

_____   _____

Do not worry if all the blanks are not filled in.

I recommend that you take the time and return to this exercise periodically as new experiences will arise. This is a great way to not only keep your self-esteem healthy but also to remind you of all you have to be grateful for and how much you have grown.

Finally, this is an "all age" exercise. This is an especially good exercise for young children. Even if they can't read or write, you can ask them these questions and let them answer. What a way to build an amazing foundation for healthy self esteem!

Test: Self-Help Reflections
(For Certification)

Requirements:

Please answer the question on a *separate sheet(s) of paper*. For certification purposes include the following:

- **Your name**
- **Date you are completing this test**
- **Write/type out the question and the answer.**

Write at least one page.

1.   What was your experience working through the self-help section (was it beneficial, confusing, difficult, etc.) Feel free to write out all your thoughts openly and honestly.

Your thoughts will not be judged and will be kept confidential. Keep a copy for yourself, it will be shredded after reviewing it to protect your right to privacy.

Even if you are not seeking certification, it would still be of great benefit to you to write out your reflections.

Chapter 3

The Energy Fields

"The most beautiful thing we can experience is the mysterious.
It is the source of all true art and science"
ALBERT EINSTIEN

Introduction to Energy Fields

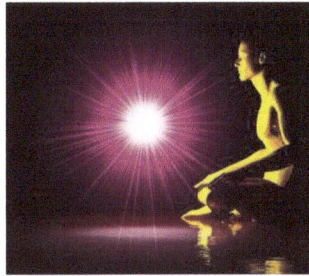

Now that you have completed all the exercises and hopefully embraced the process and gained from it, we will begin the healing arts course. This book builds chapter by chapter. It's in a particular order for a reason. That first chapter delves into the very core of who you are and why you're on this journey. It is the foundation to be laid and built upon. Without that, the rest is just smoke and mirrors. As you begin to nurture the healer within, you will have fascinating revelations. From these, you can derive knowledge that will enable you to become a better healer.

Working with Energy

Physical shifts

As you begin to work with the energy fields of the body (Chi and Chakras) you may find that you have a cold or flu, or that you have unusual aches and pains. This is because the energy state that your mind and body have become accustomed to are shifting and realigning as toxins are being released. Old fears, angers or issues may resurface. They may not be obvious or recognized for what they are. They will instead manifest as physical ailments like a cold or flu. This is a *good* thing! It means that you are successfully moving the energy to a higher vibration, a healthier level. Do not be discouraged, it will pass. As time goes on, you may experience this again on deeper levels. All this is a natural progression, part and parcel if you will, of becoming a healer. The following pages will take you through the ins and outs of energy and how it works.

Julie Bradshaw, author of the 2nd book in our series shares this story. "In one of my Celtic Shamanism classes in Ireland there was a woman who had attended quite a few seminars and was working her way into the healing arts. At this particular meeting she was feeling quite stuck. This happens to us all at one time or another. By the close of the weekend-long seminar this exchange took place between her and our teacher.

Bernie: "Well, I'll tell ya, I was about fed up with all this! I got so angry and frustrated that I just wasn't seeing anything happen. So I said, 'God, if you just show me, I'll believe it. Show me or I'm walking away and leaving it behind me!'"
Martin: "Well, that's the funny thing about Spirit. Spirit says 'Believe it and I'll show you!'"

We all had a good laugh about that and the student did agree that she had come to just that conclusion. She let it go and believed. All sorts of wonderful things opened up for her after that."

Spirit is everywhere and the energy that moves through it moves through everyone and everything. Believe it!

WHAT IS CHI?

Our ancestors, living a lifestyle void of all the distractions of today were keenly sensitized to energies below, above and around them; even within themselves. Those living closely with the vibrations of nature are more attuned to their own natures and are therefore more aware of their own physical condition on a regular basis, as well as, perhaps, addressing their needs more readily.

For example: they could feel what we know today as negative ions eliciting a state of peace. They learned through experience that they felt better near a waterfall, stream, ocean or forest. Some of these areas became sacred places to them. We know today that where there is a concentrated area of negative ions, our bodies respond with relaxation and our brain waves shift to an alpha/meditative state. However, modern man has created a split between the body and nature; between the inner and outer self.

They knew what we are only beginning to re-discover: that energy around us interacts with energy within us and vice versa and that there is no separation. Unity, inter-connectiveness to the earth, sky and each other is ultimately what keeps us healthy and whole. Being in a state of wellness or well-being is being in a state where our physical, mental, emotional and spiritual facets are not in separation but in a balanced unity, much like a balanced mobile.

A hanging mobile has a number of parts balancing nicely and returning to balance after the wind shifts it. If you take away any one of it's parts, the mobile can no longer balance itself. In our distracted, noisy, busy world, we too often ignore or devalue our needs to be whole; too much thinking and not enough feeling; too physical and not enough reflection and so on. Every facet of ourselves has significance to our health.

Everything we are is formed from and maintained by energy. In India, this energy, or life force, is called "Prana". The Chinese call it "Chi". The Japanese call it "Ki". In the Jewish Kabbalah, it is termed "The astral light". Christians call it "The Breath of God" and it is this which is used for faith healings given by priests and ministers. They are the conduit between God's life force and the patron. As a healer you, too, are a conduit.

Nearly every culture at some time recognizes the energy field emanating from all living things. So this is not "New Age" thinking. This is "Old Age" thinking, whose wisdom came from thousands of years of experience. Today, more and more scientific findings and theories are explaining the nature and interaction of energy. Beliefs that were once considered mystical and dismissed are now becoming possibilities and even probabilities.

The breath of life, Chi, is energy becoming matter and continues to exist as matter becomes Chi. As we all know, energy cannot be created or destroyed. It just changes. At the subatomic level, *our Chi is changed by what we do, say, think, feel and ingest.*

We must be cognizant of our needs. A body-mind split cannot, by the laws of nature, maintain health. None of us can be perfect. It is simply a goal towards healing and longevity.

SOURCES OF CHI

The three primary sources of Chi.

1. ***Innate Chi:*** The amount of energy we are born with. Some babies are born with an abundance of energy and (unless an illness occurs) carry that high energy into adulthood. Other babies are born with less Chi and are often tired or mellow in temperament and activity. This is their nature, just as some plants thrive more than others. It's just the way it is.

2. ***Ingested Chi:*** We receive Chi through "live" food: fruits, vegetables, nuts, etc.

3. ***Outside Chi:*** We receive more Chi directly from the environment in the form of the four basic elements; air, water, fire and earth. Our natural surroundings emit life-force which can be harnessed, intermingling with our own life-force, through spending time in nature and conducting exercises outdoors, such as Tai Chi and Yoga, both of which emphasize mind/body/breath unity.

4. I will add a fourth source: ***Prayer and Meditation***
    Because we are a microcosm of the universe, when we are praying (talking) or meditating (listening), we are expanding our consciousness to re-unite with the parent source life-force. It doesn't matter what you call it, whether astral travel or visiting God. The point is, our energies are united with the source and we are being fed.

In summary, it is important that all of the above sources of Chi are acknowledged first, acted upon next. Keep it simple. Aristotle said, "Moderation, unto all things, moderation". The Chinese express a similar philosophy: "When it is enough, stop". In other words, more is not better.

As a healer, you will be channeling from the basic Chi source. Again, call it God or the universe, it's all the same. It is, in essence, Harmony.

Exercises
To Feel Chi

1) Sit comfortably and take a few deep breaths. Now, lift your hands in front of you with your palms facing each other as if you are holding a ball of light. You may feel heat or tingling in your palms. Next, widen the space between your hands as if holding a bigger ball and slowly bring your palms closer together. Widen the space even more and repeat. See if you can feel the differences in density in the different sizes. With time, you will become more sensitive to the vibrational differences.

Don't be discouraged if you never feel energy. I have had many students who were never able to do so but were great healers, nonetheless. These students' works are testimonials for the term "faith healing".

2) Have a partner sit facing you. You are both knee to knee. Have your partner place his hands comfortably on his lap with his palms up towards the sky. Now, place your palms about 2" above his, then 4", then 6", then 1', then 2'. Slowly raise and lower your palms to feel the ball of Chi just as you did in the above exercise. You will find that both of you will experience the sensations. Next, switch places and repeat the exercise.

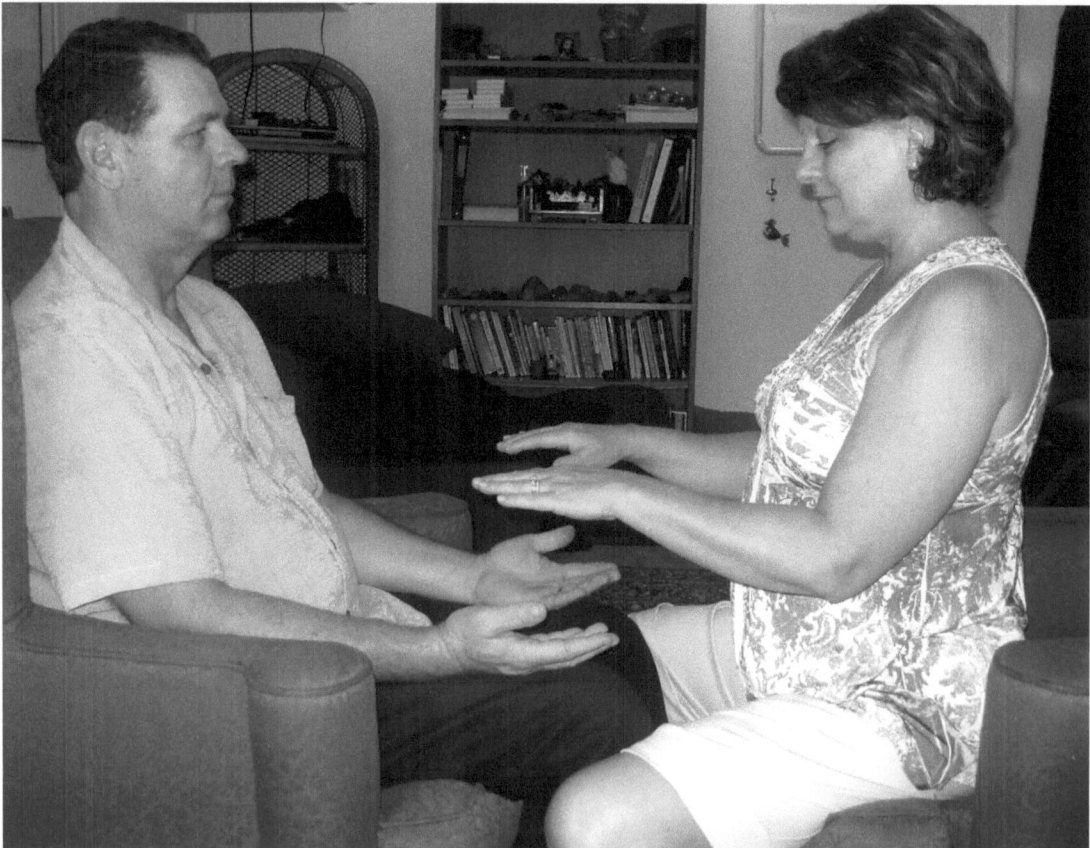

"Feeling the Chi"

The Aura

Have you ever felt the presence of someone standing behind you? Have you ever felt uncomfortable when someone was standing too close to you, like in the checkout line at the grocery store? Imagine an invisible bubble around you containing all of your energy. How far out does it extend? 2'? 3'? More?. When someone is standing within that bubble, you feel it. This is your "aura" and the size of it is your natural "auric boundary".

Everyone's comfort zone is different, but a 3' auric boundary is common. That's for us "normies". Those committed to a life of prayer and meditation have auras extending much farther and wider. For example, when I saw the Dalai Lama in a large auditorium, his aura filled the room.

Webster's defines an aura as:

1. a subtle sensory stimulus.
2. a distinctive atmosphere surrounding a given source ("the place had an aura of mystery")
3. a luminous radiation: a nimbus
4. an energy field that is held to emanate from a living being.

In the following Polaroid photos taken in 1995 & 1996, you can see differences in my aura. Note: because the auric field is three dimensional and in constant motion, orbiting around the body, the specific colors of each chakra are often not seen in their expected locations. Also, a block or upset in a chakra will result in a different color being exhibited.

Every couple of months, I would have an "imaging aura photo" taken and log my activities and state of mind at the time of the photo. As you can see, my energy field reflected my moods and the changes in them.

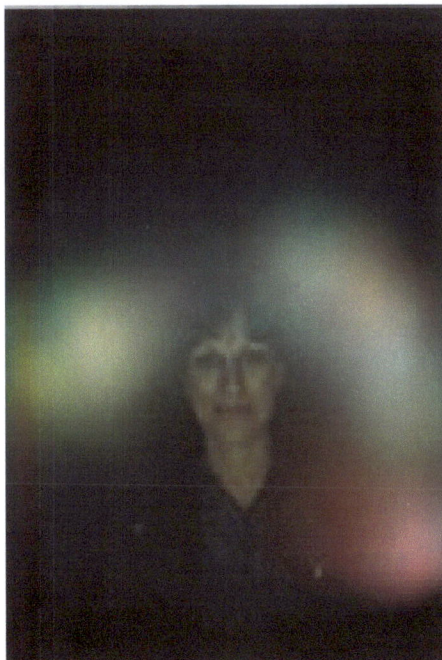

1.) Fatigue, depression, grief, not eating, closed heart chakra and crown chakra, (experienced the death of a dear friend at this time).

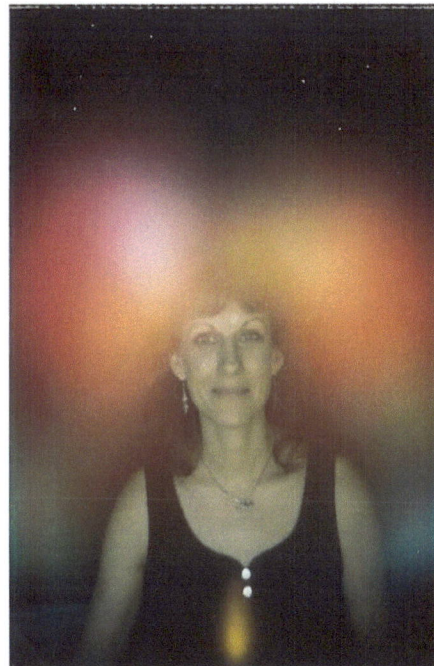

2.) Physical (red) energy coming back, some anger (red), heart chakra opening, crown chakra still closed-disconnected to God.

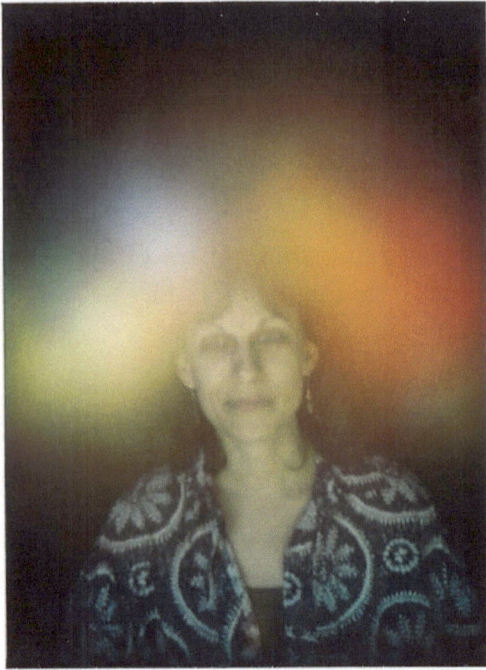

3.) Nearly balanced aura. Crown chakra is muddy as it starts to open up. I am healing, regaining faith and meditation practice.

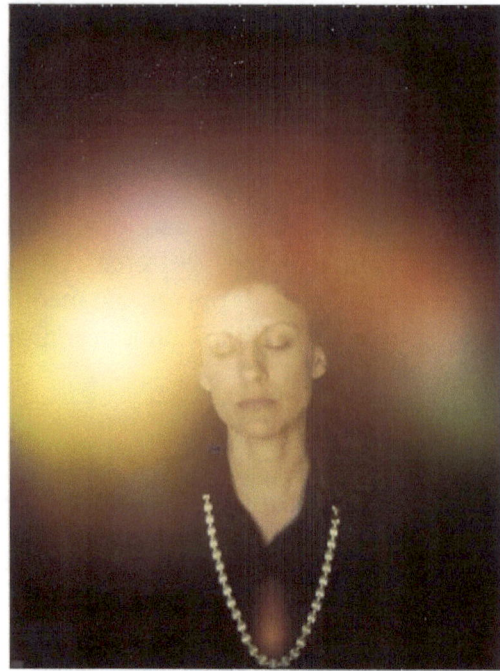

4.) Not a balanced aura. Very busy in work (red) and mental preoccupation (yellow); Beta brain waves.

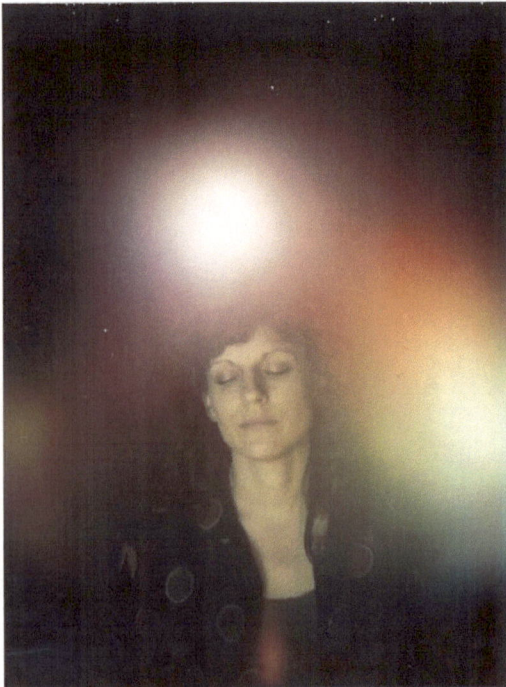

5.) Full balanced aura. Crown Chaka wide open. I was praying when this photo was taken.

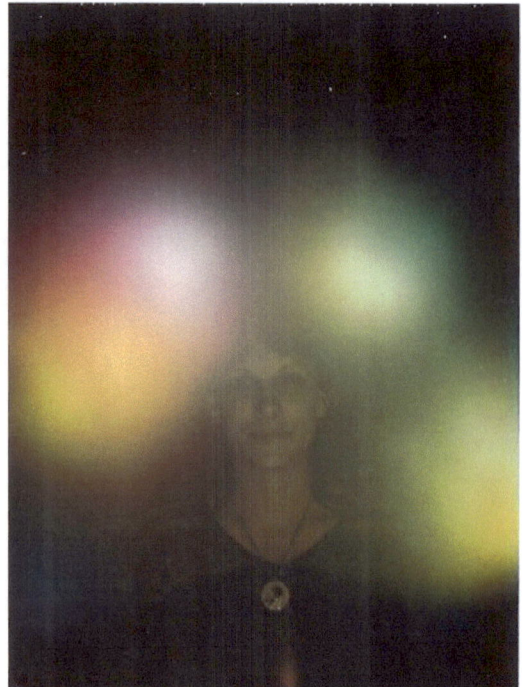

6.) Mentally busy (yellow). Tired (low red) but heart and crown chakras are open. I was teaching and counseling a lot that week.

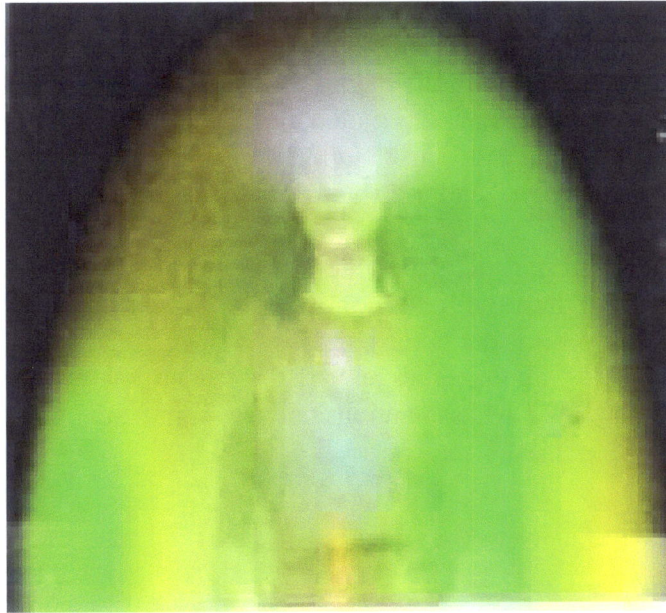

7.) Full and balanced. Third eye (blue violet) wide open. All the other chakras open as well. Green (Love) is dominant because I had just finished doing a healing.

The aura is a projection of radiant, luminous energy into the space surrounding the body in all directions, similar to the sun. This field of energy, resembling the one surrounding our planet, flows clockwise north of the equator and counterclockwise south of the equator. This is called the Coriolis effect: the rotation of fluids and gases on a rotating body (in this case, Earth).

The human body consists primarily of fluids (approx. 73%) in the same ratio as water to land on the earth. Because of this, we are subject to the Coriolis effect. We call this field the "human energy field" or "aura".

Our auric field flows down the right side and up the left side of our human body (clockwise) if we live north of the equator. If you visit Australia, the reverse is true (it's not just jet lag you are experiencing). You can verify this by watching the direction of water flow when you flush the toilet.

Recalling that Chi becomes matter, life consists of four states of matter: liquid, solid, gas and plasma. Fire and electricity are plasmas, having mass and volume, both of which constantly change. Pulses, waves, frequencies, vibrations, electromagnetism, thermal, sonic and visual stimuli are all forms of energy changing continuously.

These changes in and of the fields are also influenced by thoughts, feelings, physical phenomena, illness, temperature, elements and other external frequencies. Negative people, places and things can directly affect you when in close proximity.

You could eventually pick up someone's negativity if you're with them long enough. I've had students who would pick up or take in their client's headache or joint pain. This is called "sympathetic" or "empathic merging" and is obviously something to avoid. All of us are merging auras throughout the day. As a healer, however, this merging is of an intimate, energetic nature and it is imperative that the healer cleanse and ground after a healing, restoring her own auric boundary.

The Auric Layers

Notice on the next page, the aura has 4 distinctive layers. The first layer emanates from the lower chakras, the most dense in coalesced energy. This is called the "physical" aura, extending approx. 4" from the body and is the easiest to feel with the palms. The second layer emanates from the mid-chakras, which are less dense in vibration and is called the "emotional" aura. The third layer emanates from the upper chakras, still less dense in vibration and is called the "mental" aura. The fourth aura emanates from the "3rd eye" and crown chakra, least dense of all and is called the "spiritual" aura.

Our body, mind, emotions and spiritual experiences are imprinted and expressed throughout the aura. Illness most often begins in the auric field. For example, clinical/severe depression begins in the spiritual, emotional/mental aura. If it is not taken care of, it will eventually become matter on the physical level as a physical illness. Cancer takes approx. 10 years to materialize in the body. In a later chapter, we will go into the details of the associations between mind and body, as well as discussing cellular memory.

Spiritual

Mental

Emotional

Physical

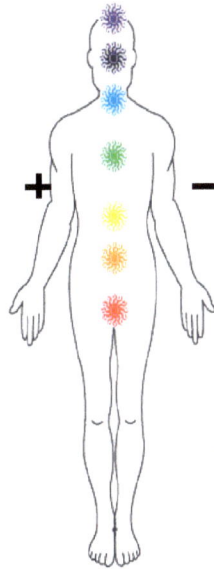

+ −

4-6" from the body

10" from the physical body

20" from the physical body

Undefined/Etheral

67

Now *you* color it!

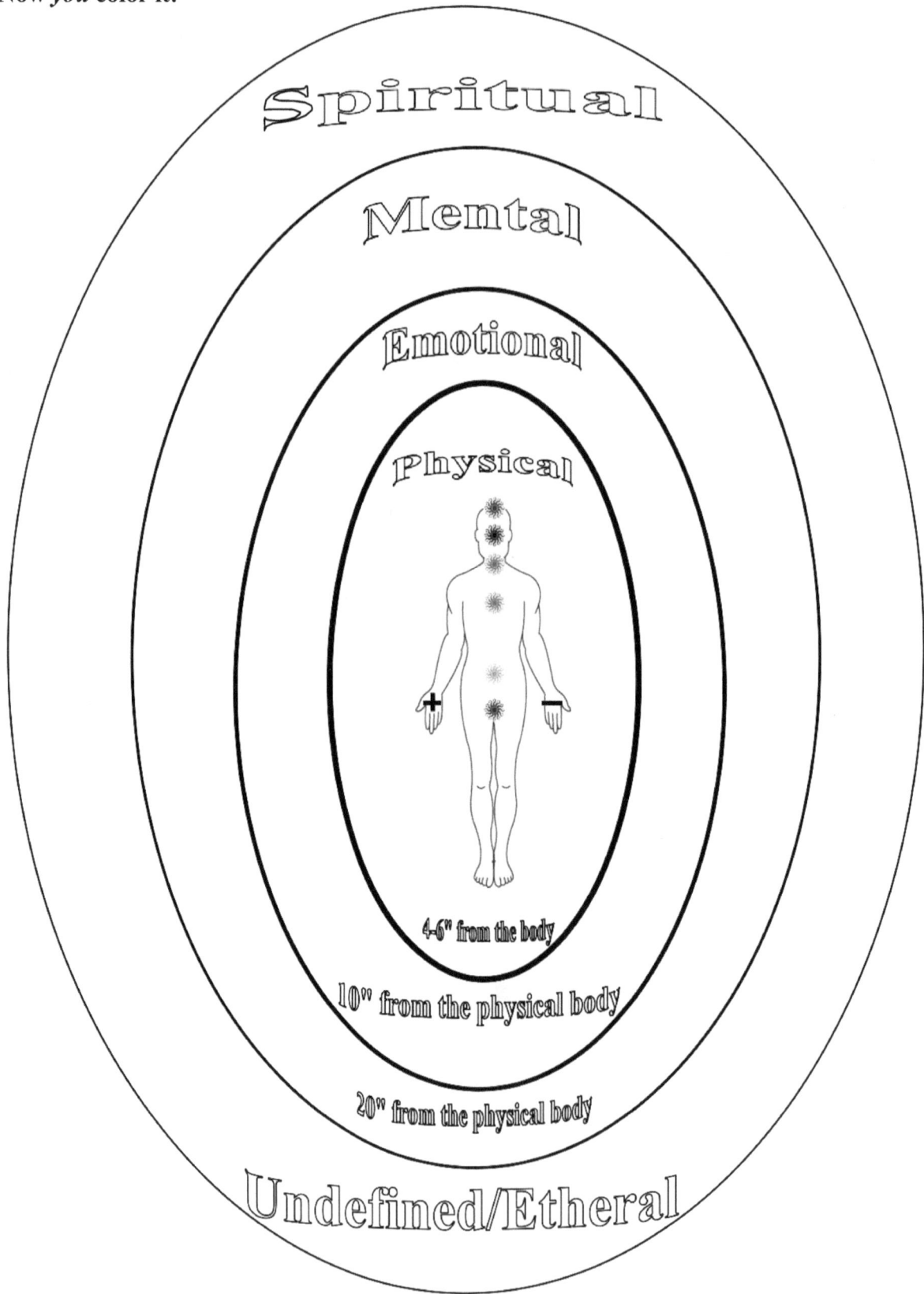

Spiritual

Mental

Emotional

Physical

4-6" from the body

10" from the physical body

20" from the physical body

Undefined/Etheral

Aura Sense Exercises

Once in a while, I can see a person's aura. (Some people have an innate ability to do this.) Artists, sensitives and right-brain people seem to have the ability to see or sense energy. There are many Christian paintings that depict a "halo" of light above the head of a saint or other sacred figures. This is the light shining from the crown chakra. These paintings sometimes also show a glowing light radiating around the whole figure. This is the aura. Would an artist paint this if it were not witnessed?

Exercise 1: Have someone stand in front of a very light or very dark wall. As you stand facing them, squint your eyes and slightly cross them so that you are using your peripheral vision more so than looking straight ahead. You may see a color or waves of energy (like heat waves from a car) around their figure.

Exercise 2: Have a partner sit in front of a mirror with their eyes closed. Stand behind them and place your palms 2 feet above their head (above the crown chakra). Slowly lower your palms until your partner senses the presence of your hands and says "stop". Repeat this several times until the "stop" level is confirmed. Keep your hands at that level and have your partner open their eyes to also confirm the distance. You are now both feeling your partner's aura.

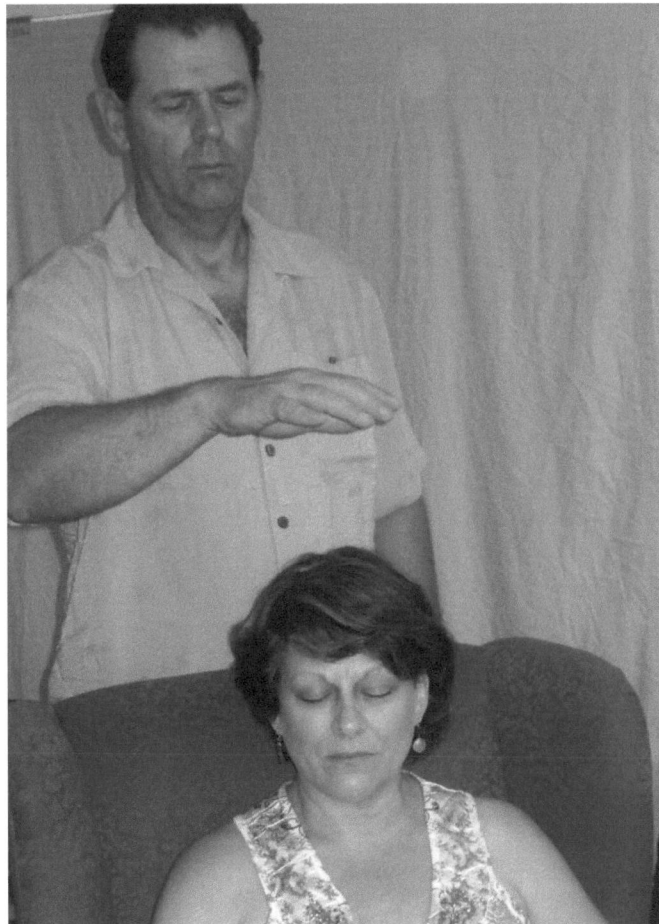

Exercise 2- Sensing the Aura

69

Scanning the Aura

1. Have your client lie down on a healing table. Use your most sensitive palm (with practice you will know which one) and very slowly sweep down their physical aura (4" to 6" away) from forehead to ankles. You want to focus on the texture and density of the energy you sense: smooth, light, thick, rough. Sweep again and this time focus on temperature: hot or cold localized spots. Sweep again focusing on unevenness: peaks or troughs. You are looking for anomalies in an otherwise smooth flowing surface.

2. Scan the joints and organ areas using the same procedure. With practice, you will be surprised at how adept you can become, feeling all these anomalies. I once scanned over a clients knee and felt a bumpy, hot sensation. I asked him if he was having any trouble with that knee. He said that he had had surgery on it for a torn ligament a couple of years ago (old injuries can remain imbalanced for quite awhile). If a client answers "no" to such a question, it is of no concern. You are probably just feeling fluctuations of energy.

There are a few hot spots which are common in people. You will often feel the liver area as hot. You can ask if they have any liver or gallbladder problems, but most of the time they won't. These organs work hard detoxifying the body and are, at times, overloaded, which causes them to emit heat.

Do not ever scare a client by diagnosing a health problem. When you feel an anomaly, you can ask "I'm just wondering if you have any concerns in this area?" If they say no but then inquire as to why are you asking, answer them with assurance: "Not to worry, it's just a movement of energy.", or "It's just a little inflamed here." Always stay positive. Remember you are not a doctor.

3. After you have scanned the physical aura, scan the emotional aura (10" above body). This is a finer vibrational frequency and not as easy to feel at first. It took me years to become sufficiently sensitized. Knowing that chronic illness starts in the emotional/mental fields, these anomalies can tell you a lot. Until you have a trusting history with a client, it is best to keep what you think you find to yourself. This arena is a therapist's job. (In a later series, we will cover mind/body dialogue which is the best way for a client to discover for themselves the emotional and mental causes of their condition.)

However, as a healer, you can work on the auric level to begin removing blocks, awaken your client's awareness and restore the meridian flows. A healing is not limited to the physical body. Clients issues will be stirred up with healings. They may deflect or ignore it because they are not ready to face it. That's okay. Again, never push the river. This is their journey in their time, not yours.

Test: Energy Fields
(For Certification)

Requirements:

Please answer each question on a *separate sheet(s) of paper*. For certification purposes include the following:

- Your name
- Date you are completing this test
- Write/type out each question, then answer it.

1. How would you explain "Chi" to a new client?

2. What are the 4 sources of Chi?

3. How would you explain the "Aura" to a new client?

4. Name the 4 layers of the aura.

5. Which is the densest layer and easiest to feel?

6. What direction does the auric field rotate North of the equator?

7. Why is this important to know in regards to a healing?

8. Approximately how far out does the physical aura extend from the body?

9. Approximately how wide in diameter does the auric field extend around the entire body?

10. What occurs when an electron is not observed by the eye and then is observed?

11. What does this imply in terms of energy and thought?

12. In an auric photo, why do some chakra colors seem to be out of place (not in their proper location)?

13. What are you looking for when scanning an aura?

14. What organ will often feel hot because it is commonly over-worked?

15. What do you think a client would feel if you were to smudge against their auric flow directions?

16. If a client gets a cold or experiences emotional discomfort after a healing, what does this mean?

What is a Chakra?

Chakras are simply loci of focused energy, both producing and receiving Chi. Energy enters from the top crown chakra and anchors at the root chakra. (We die from the feet up and leave the body through the crown). Chakras absorb universal Chi energy into the body, which then nourishes all bodily systems, including the internal organs, the nervous system, the endocrine glands, the circulatory system, etc.

The body stores Chi, especially in the 2nd chakra (which I call the "storage tank"). Indian yoga calls it the "Hara"; the Chinese call it the "Dan Tien". This chakra is extremely vulnerable to prolonged illness. It is akin to a water reservoir and, if drained too much, the body can start declining and dying. This storage tank needs to be kept full. Any excess Chi flows, or circulates, along the meridians (Yoga term: Nadis). *Always give this chakra extra Chi in a healing.*

I compare the chakras to the wiring system in a house. Electrical wiring always connects at some point. That point of connection is the chakra of our electrical system. Since a chakra is a focalized spot, it will appear as a focalized spot of light. Chakras look like cones or spirals of light originating from the inside, shining outward through both the front and back of the body. Because they are localized, they are denser and easier to feel with the hands than the general aura is.

Each chakra point correlates with each of the glands. Ancient man's observations through sensations recognized these pulsating vortexes of life-force within the body. Today, we know them as the endocrine system. Chinese medicine considers this hormonal system the essential foundation for the immune system.

The glands produce enzymes and hormones, both of which are vital sources of the body's energy and sources of change in all other systems of the body. When one gland is problematic, all the others are affected. The endocrine system (the chakra totem) is a complex system of interconnected glandular activity, often working overtime to stay balanced. Like any energy source, therefore, these chakra locations need recharging to continue to produce energy.

Colors of the Chakras

We have all seen the beauty of the rainbow spectrum. Each band of light reflects one specific color. Each color represents a different wavelength and frequency of light. The longer the wavelength, the lower the frequency and the redder the light that is produced. Conversely, the shorter and faster the wavelength, the higher the frequency, the most energetic and the bluer the light that is produced.

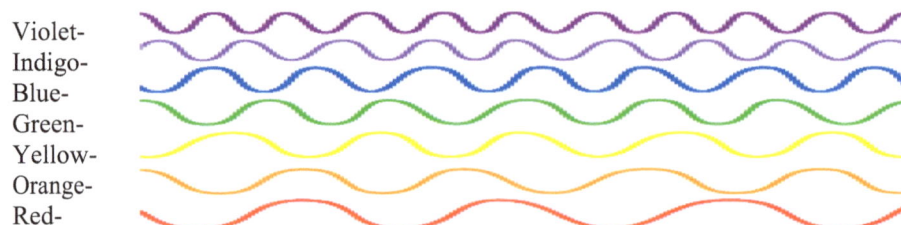

We call this the "difference in density" when scanning the chakra. The root chakra is red and thus denser and easier to feel. The crown chakra is white, lighter in density thus more difficult to feel. Our chakra totem reflects the same bands of light as the rainbow. If you could imagine seeing beyond our physical form, you would be seeing the "light body" which is as beautiful as the rainbow.

Each chakra's frequency also carries particular aspects of our consciousness, which will be explained in a later chapter. The basic correlations between human experiences and each chakra are described on the next page.

Chakra Properties: *Scanning the Chakra Totem*

Scan each chakra first in the physical, then in the emotional aura, as you did when scanning the overall aura. Again, look for variances in texture, density and evenness.

If the energy level of the heart chakra of a client is too low but the energy level of the 2nd chakra is too high, then the energy block is in the solar plexus region. If you dam a river, one side of the dam will be full while the other side of the dam will be somewhat depleted. In this client's case, you will want to focus on removing the obstruction of flow which is in the solar plexus. This process will be explained in a later chapter as well.

Practice scanning chakras with as many people as you can. Only with practice can you become sensitized to the subtlety of different frequencies and vibrations of energy.

CROWN CHAKRA

Location/Governs: Crown of the head

Color: Light Violet to White

The Center of: Collective consciousness; connection with Universe/Higher Power

Emotions: Bliss, freedom, wholeness

Gland: Pineal

Gem: Rose Quartz, Fluorite, Rose Quartz

Sound: Om-NG

Essential Oils: Lavender, Frankincense

Mantra: "I am divine" "I am beauty"

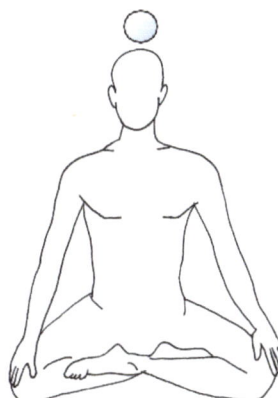

BROW CHAKRA (Third Eye)

Location/Governs: The atlas; third eye

Color: Blue Violet

The Center of: E.S.P.; dream world, insight

Emotions: Faith, confident, knowledge

Gland: Pituitary

Gem: Amethyst, Sapphire

Sound: Om

Essential Oils: Lavender, Sandalwood

Mantra: "I know my Truth" "I am guided"

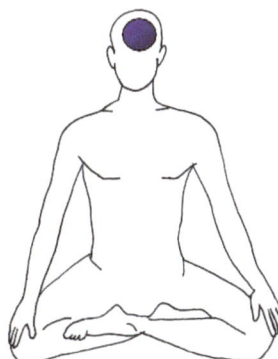

THROAT CHAKRA

Location/Governs: Third cervical; throat

Color: Blue to Sky Blue

The Center of: Speaking your truth self-expression; creativity

Emotions: Joy, relief, freedom

Gland: Thyroid

Gem: Turquoise, Lapis, Blue Kyanite

Sound: HAM

Essential Oils: Peppermint, Spruce, Thyme, Cinnamon, Nutmeg

Mantra: "I am free to be creative and expressive"

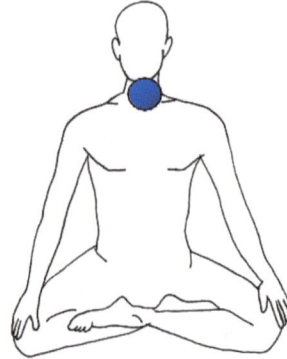

HEART CHAKRA

Location/Governs: First thoracic or sternum

Color: Green (pink in the Spiritual Aura)

The Center of: Center the chakra totem, balance, unconditional love

Emotions: Love, unity, compassion, forgiveness

Gland: Thymus Gland

Gem: Peridot, Jade, Malachite

Sound: YAM

Essential Oils: Lime, Eucalyptus, Camphor, Cedar

Mantra: "I am balanced. I give and receive love and compassion"

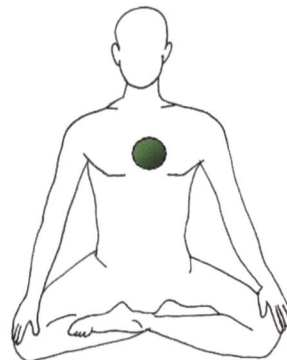

SOLAR PLEXUS CHAKRA

Location/Governs: 8th thoracic & diaphragm

Color: Yellow

The Center of: Emotions, relating with others, alarm system (butterflies in the stomach, gut feeling)

Emotions: Acceptance, patience, confidence

Gland: Pancreas

Gem: Citrine, Yellow stones, Rose Quartz

Sound: RAM

Essential Oils: Juniper, Garlic & Ginger (oral), Chamomile, Sunflower (oral), Jasmine, Lemon

Mantra: "We are all brothers and sisters on this planet home." "I am a still point in a spinning world."

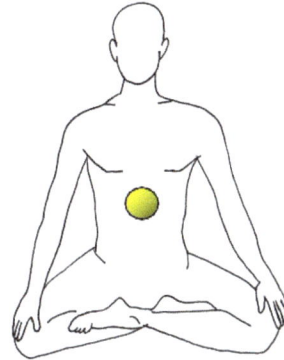

SPLEEN CHAKRA (Sacral)

Location/Governs: First lumbar, below navel

Color: Orange

The Center of: Manifestation, subconscious emotions (inner child), origin of trust/mistrust, personal growth, power spot.

Emotions: Passion, primal instincts, bonding, trust

Gland: Gonads (male testes & female ovaries)

Gem: Carnelian, Citrine, Amber, Tiger's Eye, Desert Rose

Sound: VAM

Essential Oils: Geranium, Sandalwood

Mantra: "I matter and have purpose. I am empowered."

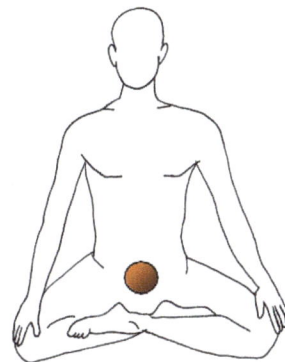

ROOT CHAKRA

Location/Governs: Genitalia, groin and coccyx

Color: Red

The Center of: Sex drive; grounding, vitality, material needs

Emotions: Feeling safe and secure, solid

Gland: Adrenal glands

Gem: Garnet, Ruby, Jasper, Onyx, Black Kyanite

Sound: LAM

Essential Oils: Clove, Pine, Sage, Patchouli

Mantra: "I am human." "I am provided for." "I am healthy."

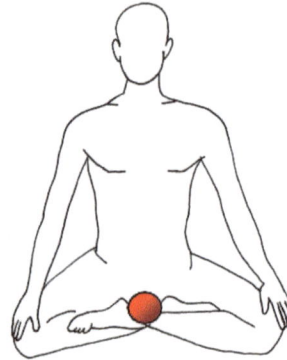

Once Upon a Time
The Chakra Story

This is the story of the journey of incarnation of the soul. Each stage of our lives encompasses a piece of this experience. We incarnate in human form to gain information, knowledge and experience and to transform them into wisdom for our souls to evolve. Of course, our journey of consciousness is not a linear progression, but intertwined, shifting with the ebbs and flows of life, interacting and repelling, but desiring forward motion, compatibility and connection with the two "I AM's": divine and human.

Rarely will you find a person that has moved forward from one level of consciousness to the next without so much as a hiccup to slow them down. We all have challenges that face us at each stage of growth. This story is a guideline that can help you understand where you are now, where you've been and where you would like to be.

Once upon a time...

You were a pure soul of the highest vibration of love and light when you were born into your human body. Your first experience of instinctual consciousness related to your root chakra. You were completely dependent on your parents to provide for all your needs, especially love and safety. *If you feel safe and are provided for, your root chakra is primarily in balance; if not, deeply ingrained fear of survival is apparent.*

As time went on, you grew as a toddler and the self-awareness related to the 2nd chakra, the *Sacral chakra. This is where trust and worthiness are defined.* You were dependent on your parents to know if you were "good enough" as a healthy relationship was being established between them and yourself. *This chakra is the most crucial for the foundation of your life. If you were not given this sense of trust and worthiness in this stage of development, your sense of personal empowerment and self-worth will be damaged and this chakra will be blocked. That is why this chakra consciousness is considered our power spot. Subconscious issues are stored here.*

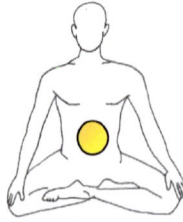

You then entered the school years and experienced the world around you. This, the *Solar plexus*, or 3rd chakra was overwhelmed with people, places and things in the outside world. You became aware of interactions with others. *If your survival needs were met in the root chakra and your self-worth was established in the sacral chakra*, your outside world will be relatively functional. *You will have a good sense of what is emotionally healthy or unhealthy. You'll have clarity and trust in your perception, the lower mind and your achieved goals. If not, the lack of self-worth will result in dysfunctional behavior. This chakra is most active on the conscious level.* Most of your lifetime will involve facing the inner conflicts and issues of the ego, identity, gut emotions, decision making, seeking and reacting. You will either choose to seek maturity or denial and addiction of some form (even chronic complaining, fear, anger, or sadness in life may become an addiction). *This is the 2nd power spot.*

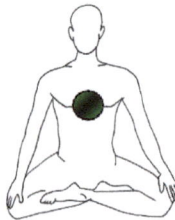

Now you've gotten older and wiser. You've gained knowledge and healthy coping skills during the lessons of life. You've achieved some goals and the goals achieved help establish self-esteem. In your maturity, you've gained understanding and compassion for others in the world outside of yourself. You've learned forgiveness and community. *This heart chakra consciousness enables you to love maturely and to be loved. If you have not taken responsibility for your growth needs, you will be stuck in a wounded child psyche, wherein this chakra will be blocked and grieving.*

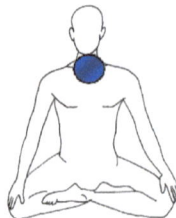

You've become more comfortable in your own skin now. You know who you are and like who you are. You continue to achieve goals and have resolved the past. You create. This *throat chakra consciousness is about freedom to speak your Truth and express yourself.* You may decide to write your book, paint, share your talents with others or volunteer. You are free to be yourself. You have a sense of inner peace and a desire to give. *If you have not developed to this level due to lack of growth, you will be utterly unfulfilled.*

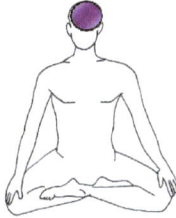

Because of this brave and enlightened journey, your consciousness has expanded. This is the higher mind: the *3rd eye chakra of greater insight.* The lower, worldly mind, the solar plexus, may be saying nothing, but your higher mind clarifies it for you. *This is the ability to know the higher Truth of your existence, the purpose of your life's walk. Meditation becomes a natural impulse elicited by a simple walk in a garden. You automatically tune into an inner guided compass.* You can see beyond this 3rd dimension at times. If you have not established this connection to your higher self, you will feel *lost, fearful* and *cynical.*

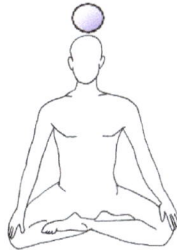

The body that was born with love and innocence, wholeness and exuberance has come full circle. *Your crown chakra is illuminated again in reunion with the source in which you came. This consciousness of the connection and eternity of all there is, all people, plants, universes, probabilities and possibilities is the ultimate release of separation.*

The crown chakra is the "I AM of God"; the root chakra is the "I AM as human."

(Never)
The End

Quite a story, isn't it? I haven't met a client or student yet who hasn't felt the impact from it, like a veil being lifted and clarity re-born. As if suddenly the dots are connected and everything makes sense. Spiritual Truth always feels this way.

So, every morning now, include 10 to 20 minutes of the Chakra Imagery followed by silent meditation on the next page. Start with just a one-week commitment.

Chakra Imagery for the Healer

To Begin

Sit comfortably. Inhale deeply 8 counts in, hold for 4 counts and release. Do this several times, releasing the stresses of the day.

Now relax your breathing and feel your body sinking heavily into your seat.

Imagine green energy coming up from the nurturing healing earth. It comes up through the soles of your feet, filling your legs and organs, all the way up the torso and back muscles and down your arms and out through your hands. It moves up into the neck and face and head. Smell the freshness of this sweet green earth as it splashes out of the crown of your head, washes down and around the aura of your entire body. and finally back down to its home beneath your feet.
Continue to breathe it in as you imagine this a few times more.

Now imagine, from above the clouds, a stream of lovely white light descending upon you, filling your entire body inside and out, flowing down and into the earth.

Relax now as you let go of the imagery. Just feel the merging of these two sources of life force. Let go of all thoughts and effort as the energies smooth out into a peaceful state. Just be at rest for a while. Take as long as you need to do this.

- Now imagine turning on the light switch of your white crown chakra. Let it shine brightly.

- Then turn on the light switch of the blue-violet 3rd eye chakra that is seeing and knowing.

- Next is the switch for the sky-blue throat chakra. Let it shine in freedom of expression.

- Breathe deeply as you switch on the green heart chakra and receive the love of the Creator.

- Now turn on the light switch of the solar plexus and let the sunshine radiate out.

- Down to the switch on the campfire orange light of the 2nd chakra. Feel the power of passion and security.

- Now, switch on the red fire of the root chakra and feel the vitality energizing every cell in your body.

- Lastly, let go of the imagery. Let your mind be free and rest in silence.

Add this step before a healing: As you breathe in with awareness of the opening and freedom of your chakra totem, feel the chair beneath you. Imagine the soles of your feet and the chakras in each palm opening to allow energy to flow out.

Closing: Let your breathing slowly return to normal as you become aware of your surroundings again.
Coming back now fully to the room, almost ready to open your eyes. Take one more deep breath, relishing the feeling of every chakra balanced and energized. Open your eyes when you're ready.

Test: Chakras
(For Certification)

Requirements:

Please answer each question on a *separate sheet(s) of paper*. For certification purposes include the following:

- **Your name**
- **Date you are completing this test**
- **Write/type out each question, then answer it.**

1. **How would you describe chakras to a new client?**

2. **What basic shape is a chakra?**

3. **Does a chakra extend out of the front of the body, the back of the body or both?**

4. **Name the 7 primary chakras and their correlating colors.**

5. **Which chakras are denser and easier to feel?**

6. **What are you looking for when scanning a chakra?**

7. **How do you determine if a chakra is blocked?**

8. **If the heart chakra feels sort of thick and the 2nd chakra feels cold or weak, where is the blockage?**

9. **Which chakra is the "Storage Tank" of Chi and needs replenishment most of the time?**

10. **What emotions, influences and mantras correlate to each of the 7 primary chakras?**

11. **After practicing the chakra imagery, which chakra(s) are you aware of that are blocked?**

Chapter 4

Mind-Body Meditations

"No one can get inner peace by pouncing on it."
HARRY EMERSON FOSDICK

How Imagery & Meditation Work

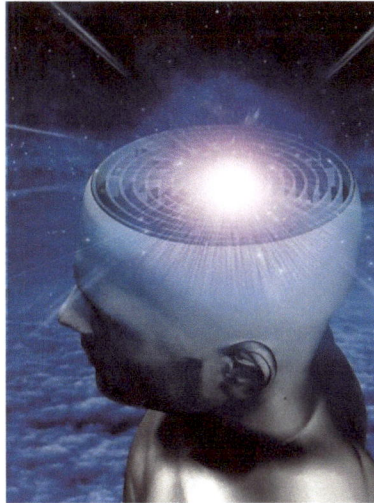

There is a vast difference between imagery and meditation. *Imagery* is visualizing people, places and things, guided orally by a healer. The most effective imageries consist of utilizing all five senses: sight, sound, smell, touch and taste (imagery that involves visualizing a place in nature). You feel the sun on your face, you smell the flowers and earth, you hear the babbling brook and see the wind move through the trees. You even taste and touch the fruit from one of those trees.

On the other hand, while *meditation* can be guided with chanting, Tibetan bowls, chimes or music and a transition to a meditative state can be made through minimal imagery (such as imagining a single candle flame), the purest form of meditation and the most challenging is sitting in silence.

That is the ultimate goal. Only in effortless silence can you meet your true and higher self. There is no phenomena, no stimuli, no outside guidance. Only in the silence can you know and harness your power of being as God's creation.

Commonly, you will sit in meditation for 45 minutes, but for only two minutes will you be "there". "There" is the moment when your expanded consciousness merges with the greater consciousness/God. You know you have been "there" when you come back "knowing" something. The "knowing" is a surety of truth for you. You are unequivocally positive of what you now "know". This is like the first time you become adept at a task, like riding a bicycle. You may not have done it for a while and be a bit shaky when you try again, but your body will remember how. Once you *know,* you can never *un*know.

What imagery and meditation have in common are positive health benefits. The immediate result of both is stress reduction because both practices shift our brain wave activity in the process. It is the most common benefit. However, the possibilities are endless: Pain relief, faster recovery from injuries, emotional healing, clarity, the experience of balance, wholeness, peace of mind and expansion of spiritual awareness.

Why Meditate?

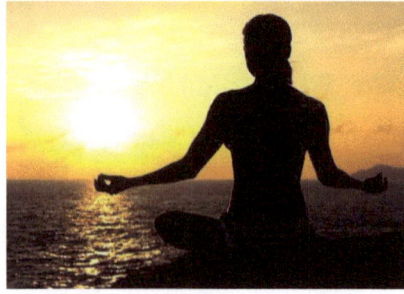

"Why do we meditate? What is it exactly? Can anyone do it? I can't get my legs in that pretzel position!" These are just a few of the questions and comments that arise when we hear the word "meditation". If you have never meditated before, understand that the brain is just another muscle in your body. If it's not used on a regular basis, it becomes out of shape, flabby. So, what is meditation and why is it important especially as a Healing Arts Practitioner?

What is meditation?

Definition: Encarta World English Dictionary
1. **emptying or concentration:** the emptying of the mind of thoughts, or the concentration of the mind on one thing, to aid mental or spiritual development, contemplation, or relaxation
2. **pondering of something:** the act of thinking about something carefully, calmly, seriously and for some time, or an instance of such thinking

We use our brains every day for thinking, reasoning and for rationalizing the mundane world around us. This is the world where we do the laundry, go to work, brush our teeth, eat, etc. The brain gets most of the exercise it needs in that respect daily and sometimes, is exhausted by it. Meditation, on the other hand, is a time to slow the mind down from the outer sensory input and discover the inner world we each house in ourselves. It is a time of peace, tranquility, quiet and connection.

Why do we meditate?

For some, it may simply be a physical practice. When you meditate, your heartbeat slows, as does your breathing and your body relaxes. There are several physical benefits to meditation. It lowers blood pressure, reduces mental and physical stress and allows more oxygen into the bloodstream, creating a valuable chain reaction in the physical body. The benefits range from healthier skin to greater nutrient absorption, as well as a myriad of other supportive functions.

Mentally and spiritually, this is a time to connect with yourself. When we take the time to meditate, we are removing ourselves from our normal lives to actively listen to our inner selves. This is our time to connect with the Divine and feed our spirit. It is a time of centering, a time of rejuvenation. You may have questions that need answering. Meditation is a great way to gain clarity for yourself and for your work with a client.

How to meditate?

There are several forms of meditation, from sitting in silence to guided imagery and even moving meditation (yoga or Tai Chi). I suggest that if you have never meditated before, a guided imagery meditation may be a good beginning. In this type of meditation, you may use a recorded CD or have someone else read the imageries and meditations offered in this book.

Guided imagery gives you a course to follow. There is a purpose, a goal to be reached. It can be physical in nature such as: learning to control breathing, release tension, reduce anxiety and pain; to energize your chakras or to visualize a better golf swing. It may be metaphorical or emotional, as in the "Tending Your Inner Garden" imagery, where you weed out and replace negative emotions or feelings that no longer serve you and symbolically plant seeds of hope and goals. Find one that feels right to you and give yourself to it completely. Remember, energy follows thought.

Silent meditation is just that, silent. There is no background music to focus on, no words to listen to. It is a very simple practice that can be a powerful experience. It is challenging especially if you live in the city. We don't realize how much background noise there is until we try to block it out. Even the quiet hum of the computer or refrigerator can be distracting but with regular practice, as you simply allow the distractions to pass by like clouds, you will discover you can meditate anywhere, anytime.

Finally, there is *moving meditation*. There are several ways to do this, from yoga, Tai Chi to walking a labyrinth painted on the ground or formed with stones, to free form dancing. Even walking around a room while concentrating on your steps is a moving meditation. You will find that if you practice for any length of time, when you move that way again, your mind will automatically shift into a meditative state.

The *pretzel pose*. It is not necessary to contort your body into inhuman shapes to meditate. Meditation may be done standing, sitting or walking. Wherever you feel most comfortable will work.

Distractions

Distractions will come from everywhere when you try to meditate. Here are some ideas to minimize them.

- Wear comfortable clothing, nothing restrictive or tight.
- Create a relaxing atmosphere with candles, lighting, aroma, or incense.
- Refrain from meditating when you're extremely hungry or after a big meal.
- Close windows and doors to minimize outside noise and neighborhood traffic.
- Unplug the phone. Turn off the cell phone.

How much? How often? What if I can't shut off my mind?

You may decide to meditate for 10 minutes and end up taking more than an hour, however, twenty minutes twice a day is the most advantageous routine.

Like exercise, it becomes easier the more you practice. If you're just starting out, you may find that silencing your inner chatter may be difficult. This is the ego that does not want to shut down. It wants attention 24/7 and will do almost anything to get it! When you find your mind wandering, simply note it and bring your attention back to whatever you've chosen to focus on for that meditation. It will get better with time so be easy on yourself.

Brain Waves Defined

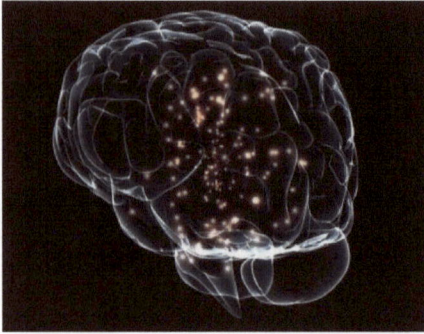
These are the neurons firing

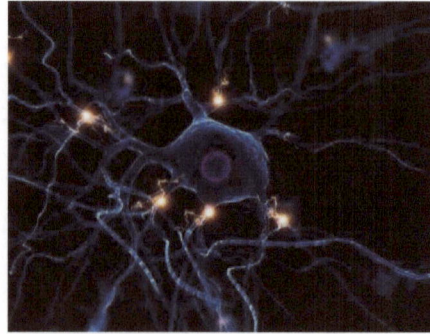
Close up of a neuron in the brain

There are several levels of brain waves. Each governs specific patterns and reactions we all have. Here are the basic stages for a healer's understanding.

- **Beta Wave:** This is our state of everyday activity. We are using our conscious mind and are awakened to all experience and stimuli around us. We experience both negative and positive stressors.

- **Alpha Wave:** When taking deep conscious breaths, relaxing and quieting ourselves, our brain waves shift to alpha. We are starting to focus inward. This state is your goal towards facilitating healings for your clients. Imageries elicit Alpha.

- **Theta Wave:** Hypnotherapy and meditation shifts the brain waves to the theta, where the conscious mind is nearly asleep, allowing the subconscious and super- conscious to emerge.

- **Delta Wave:** This is the sleep and dream state.

Alpha and theta states are essential to attain and promote body-stress and illness recovery. These are also the only states where the body itself can repair or recover energetically.

As a healer, you are inducing these states for your clients and thereby bringing them energetically into an extremely receptive state for a positive healing outcome.

Therefore, it is important for you as their healer to maintain your own alpha state during their healing.

Power of the Mind Through Imagery

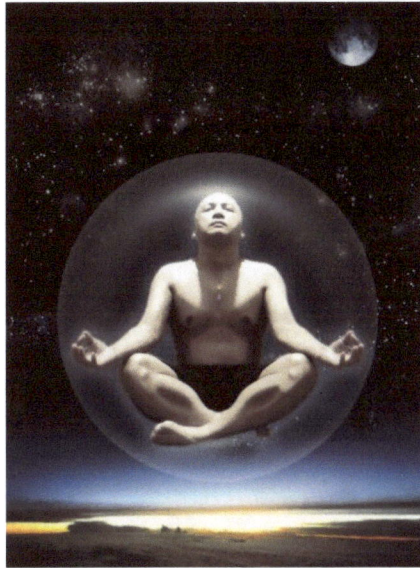

It has been said that three-fourths of healing comes from the mind. We've all heard stories of two people, both given the same diagnosis at the same time and told they have six months to live. The first dies in a month. The other lives for five more years. Why?

Attitude

Attitude plays a role and can make a difference. This is not to say that, if your attitude is spectacularly good, you'll live longer with a disease than someone with the same disease and a negative attitude. It's not that black and white. I have known folks who have gone through just the opposite. They were tremendously positive and their disease took them quickly, while others were just as negative and lived longer with the same disease. Generally however, a healthy attitude can keep your condition more stable, perhaps even slow a disease's progression.

The physical body is amazing; it has a memory of its own. Take for example the case of Mr. Christopher Reeve. After five years in a wheelchair, unable to move and on a respirator, he believed without doubt that his body would "remember" how to function.

The impact of his 215 pound (98 kg) body hitting the ground shattered his first and second vertebrae. Reeve had not been breathing for three minutes before paramedics arrived. After five days, he regained full consciousness and Dr. John Jane explained that he had destroyed his first and second cervical vertebrae, which meant that his head and spine were not connected. His lungs were filling with fluid and were suctioned by entry through the throat.

Dr. John Jane performed surgery to repair Reeve's neck vertebrae. The accident that left him a quadriplegic in 1995 did not stop him from exploring and achieving active physical rehabilitation.

In the therapy gym, Reeve worked on moving his trapezius muscle. Electrodes connected to him sent out readings to therapists and every day he would try to beat his numbers from the day before. The most difficult part of rehabilitation was respiratory therapy. The therapist, Bill Carroll, used a hose to see how much air Reeve could inhale, measured in cubic centimeters as the vital capacity. In order to even consider getting off the artificial respirator, a patient needs a vital capacity of 750 cc's.

Initially, Reeve could hardly get above zero. By the end of October, he was able to get around 50 cc's. This inspired him and he felt his natural competitive edge coming back. The next day, he went up to 450 cc's. He reached 560 cc's the day after. Bill Carroll said, "I've never seen progress like that. You're going to win. You're going to get off this thing." On December 13, 1995, Reeve was able to breathe without a ventilator for 30 minutes.

By the year 2002, after intense physical therapy and unending determination, he was able to move his index finger, breathe on his own without assistance for up to 90 minutes and feel the sensations in his body, even though it was said to be impossible. The body remembers.

Reeve has recovered to the point where he can raise his right hand to a 90-degree angle, breathe without the help of a respirator for 90 minutes at a time and distinguish between hot and cold and sharp and dull.
More importantly, Reeve says he can feel the hugs of his wife, Dana and his three children. McDonald's work with Reeve has been so impressive that it's the subject of an article in this month's Journal of Neurosurgery: Spine.
"The fact is that even if your body doesn't work the way it used to, the heart and the mind and the spirit are not diminished. It's as simple as that," said Reeve.
In November 2000, Reeve greeted his doctor, John W. McDonald, M.D., Ph.D., with a feat no one thought possible. As McDonald watched in awe, Reeve slowly and deliberately raised the tip of his left index finger. (Cited from CNN Health "Paralyzed Christopher Reeves makes slight gain." August 6, 2011)

While there is no mention of deliberate meditation on Mr. Reeve's part to prepare for the grueling physical challenge, I believe it safe to assume that he would "set his mind to the task". In doing this, simply making the choice to focus his mind in such a way is a meditation, an imagery in itself.

It is truly amazing what the human spirit and mind together may accomplish. Unfortunately, his dream of walking under his own power was not realized before he passed away from heart failure in 2004, but the work carries on. A great man, an enlightened soul, he is sorely missed.

The condition of Mr. Christopher Reeves is, of course, an extreme case. The fact that he could move some of his fingers and sense temperature is remarkable. His is one of the greatest testimonials to the power of the mind.

Can you ultimately heal dis-*ease*? Maybe not. Can you get a little better, healthier? Absolutely! I have seen it hundreds of times. One of my first teachers, Louise Taylor, told me this story. She had been asked to see a 17 year old boy who couldn't walk after a year in the hospital. Doctors basically had to put him back together after his car accident. However, they were baffled to find that even though there was no physiological reason why, he could not walk. As a last resort (holistic options often are) he was referred to Louise by a family acquaintance.

Louise saw the boy and asked him if he remembered how to walk and run. He answered "yeah". She asked him to close his eyes and remember all the things he enjoyed doing before the accident. She asked for the details of that imagery, such as what he was hearing, smelling, feeling in his memories. Lastly, when guided to open his eyes, she asked him again, "Do you remember what it was like to walk?" He answered "No, I don't".

After a few weeks of hypnotherapy and imagery sessions, he fully recovered and walked back into his life unaided. This is known as neuromuscular pathway memory.

Relaxation Imagery

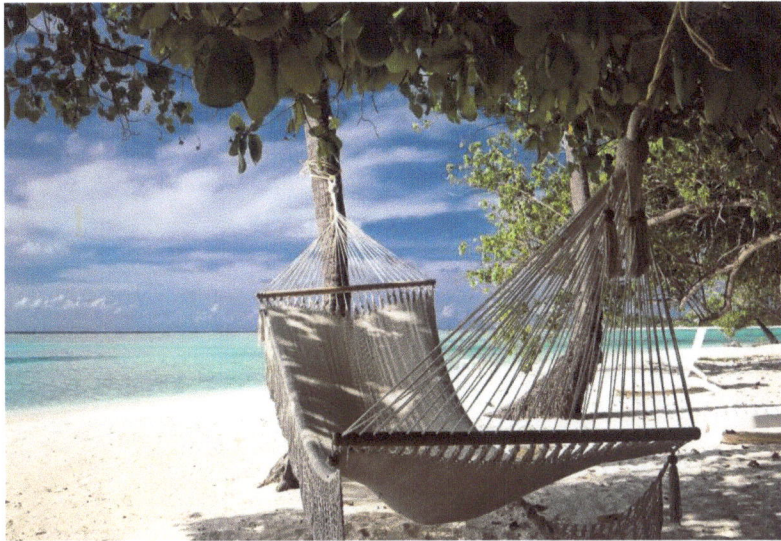

Close your eyes and take a few full, deep breaths. Imagine seeing or feeling a pink, blue, or white cloud of comfort or a warm ray of sunshine gently moving down through your skull. Let it relax the face, jaws and throat. Relax the neck, now, letting tensions melt away. Down to your right shoulder. Now the left shoulder. Let the stress simply fall off of you. Let your shoulders drop, heavy and relaxed. Let the massaging light move down and through your upper back. The middle and lower back now become heavy and relaxed, releasing even more stress and pressure. All the tightness and stress simply flows down your neck, shoulders and out the tailbone.

Now the cloud or light relaxes your right shoulder again, traveling down your forearm, leaving it heavy and relieved; the wrist and the hand, the thumb and each finger is loose and comfortable. Now the left side, from the shoulder, to the forearm again, down to the wrist, hand, thumb and each of your fingers. All the stresses flow down and out of each fingertip.

Breathe the warm light in deeply now and let it free your lungs and flow into the stomach and through the right hip. The light releases tension, down the thigh and knee to the ankle and finally the foot. All is relaxed and calm with one deep exhale.

Breathe the cloud or light in one more time from the lungs into the stomach and let it flow into your left hip, down the thigh, through the knee to the ankle and out the foot. Deep inhale, deep exhale. Your entire body is heavy. You are free. Rest, relax and enjoy as long as you want. (Note: Rest quietly for a few minutes before proceeding with any added-on imageries or meditations.)

Closing:
Let your breathing slowly expand as you become aware of your surroundings again. Coming back now fully to the room almost ready to open your eyes. Take in a refreshing breath of life force, relishing the feeling of complete relaxation. Open your eyes when you're ready.

Nature Imagery

This imagery may be used by itself or directly after the Relaxation Imagery. They work together wonderfully to center yourself after a difficult day or to prepare for one. This is also a great daily practice to stimulate the pleasure center of the brain which elicits optimism, as well as, stimulating the cellular healing processes due to the wholistic interplay with the 5 senses.

Let's begin:

Imagine going to your favorite place in nature. You find a serene place to sit or lie down. Breathe in deeply as you relax from head to toe. Feel the sunlight or soft breeze on your face, your skin, so warming and comforting. Breathe it into your lungs and then your whole body. It feels so good, nourishing you completely.

Notice now the beautiful blue sky above you and lush greens around you. You can smell the clean rich aroma of earth and water. Breathe it all in as the stress just melts off of you.

As you let the sunlight or breeze massage into every muscle, feel the ground under your feet and all of nature around you, healing you. Soak it all up like a sponge (the blue sky, sounds of the nearby water, the birds, the light, the scenery, the aromas).

Now imagine picking a lovely piece of fruit that is growing on the tree next to you. The texture is wonderful and the smell is sweet and clean. You take a bite of this juicy fruit. It is like nothing you've ever tasted, so perfect and you feel its nutrients feeding your entire body. Every cell is refreshed, rejuvenated. Relax and enjoy this feeling and space as long as you like…

Now, see yourself standing up amidst this beautiful place, stretching and smiling, feeling refreshed and strong, knowing all is well.

Closing:

Let your breathing slowly expand as you become aware of your surroundings again. You are coming back now fully to the room, almost ready to open your eyes. Take one more deep breath, relishing the feeling of lightness and joy. Open your eyes when you're ready.

Pain Reduction Imagery

This imagery helps to reduce aches and pains in the physical body whether it is a chronic pain or from a recent injury. They are all a dis-*ease* physically manifested in the body. Always start with the Relaxation Imagery before any pain reduction technique.

Let's begin:

1. Close your eyes and check your physical level from 1 to 10 (10 being the most pain; 1 being completely pain free and relieved). What number are you? *Record this on the log sheet later.*

2. Start with *Relaxation Imagery,* then follow with…

Pain Reduction Imagery

Now, go to your favorite place in nature and find the perfect spot to rest. Next to you is a shallow pool or vessel of some kind, filled with healing, sparkling cold water and ice.

Imagine seeing the area of your pain as fiery red and inflamed. Lower this body part in the cold ice water. If your whole body hurts, then float in the cool shallow pool. If you cannot get that particular body part in the water, use a cup, ladle or your hand to scoop up the water and pour it on the afflicted area. Know that whatever you need will be readily at hand. Let the cold penetrate into the red inflamed pain, easing it, cooling it. The red is fading now, being replaced by the blue tint in the healing waters as it dissolves all the inflammation.

Breathe in cool blue for three counts, 3, 2, 1. Then breathe out *total relief* at 0. Exhale forcefully and release all pain. Continue until the redness has completely disappeared and has been replaced by the blue sparkling color.

Now relax your breathing. Your entire being is radiating soft pastel colors of the rainbow. Relax even deeper now. Enjoy this peaceful state as long as you want…

Closing:
Let your breathing slowly expand as you become aware of your surroundings again. You are coming back now to the room, ready to open your eyes, feeling refreshed.

3. Check in from 1 to 10 again. Record the number on the log sheet. Did your level of pain go down or is it same?

The more often you practice this exercise, the greater the positive results. It takes time to train the brain to send these messages to the body. Use this technique as often as you can. I recommend you do it every day for at least 10 minutes.

You will only get out of it what you put into it. Be patient and committed. It may take weeks or months until you feel results. This is why it is important to log your check-ins. Even the smallest change is a positive one. The mind is an amazing, complex computer and the body will eventually respond to this specific data input. Yes, you *can* train your *brain- to- body* responses.

Log Sheets for Pain Reduction

Date	Day	Pain Level Before	Pain Level After
1/1/11	1	10	10
1/2/11	2	10	9
1/3/11	3	9	9
1/4/11	4	9	8
1/5/11	5	9	8
1/6/11	6	9	8
1/7/11	7	8	8
1/8/11	8	8	7
1/9/11	9	7	7
1/10/11	10	7	7
1/11/11	11	7	4
1/12/11	12	6	5
1/13/11	13	5	5
1/14/11	14	5	5
1/15/11	15	5	4

Date	Day	Pain Level Before	Pain Level After
1/16/11	16	5	4
1/17/11	17	4	4
1/18/11	18	4	4
1/19/11	19	4	4
1/20/11	20	4	3
1/21/11	21	4	3
1/22/11	22	3	3
1/23/11	23	3	3
1/24/11	24	3	2
1/25/11	25	3	2
1/26/11	26	3	2
1/27/11	27	2	2
1/28/11	28	2	1
1/29/11	29	1	1
1/30/11	30	0	0

Pain Levels	
1	No pain to very mild
2	No pain to very mild
3	No pain to very mild
4	Moderate
5	Moderate
6	Moderate
7	Moderate to severe
8	Moderate to severe
9	Moderate to severe
10	Moderate to severe

Column 1: The date of your meditation.
Column 2: Keeping track of the days.
Column 3 & 4: Recording your pain levels before and after your meditations.

Several lines for notes have also been included. If you skip a day, make a note as to why or what happened. This history will help in reviewing your progress from this exercise.

Daily Check In Log Sheets

Date	Day	Pain Level Before	Pain Level After
	1		
	2		
	3		
	4		
	5		
	6		
	7		
	8		
	9		
	10		
	11		
	12		
	13		
	14		
	15		

Date	Day	Pain Level Before	Pain Level After
	16		
	17		
	18		
	19		
	20		
	21		
	22		
	23		
	24		
	25		
	26		
	27		
	28		
	29		
	30		

Pain Levels	
1=	
2=	No pain to very mild
3=	
4=	
5=	
6=	Moderate
7=	
8=	
9=	Moderate to severe
10=	

Notes: _____
_____
_____
_____
_____
_____
_____
_____
_____
_____
_____
_____
_____
_____

Deep Meditation

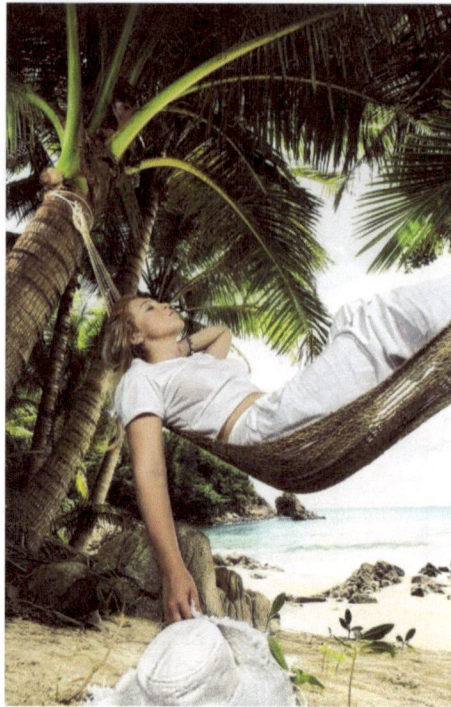

This meditation will allow you to shift into the twilight between asleep and awake, a state in which you may reach the theta brain wave (deepest state of relaxation). When you are finished, you will be refreshed as if you took a rejuvenating nap.

To begin, you may wish to distract the mind chatter and prepare for a deeper level of meditation by using soft music. Limit the time to one or two tracks rather than the whole CD. This will allow for time in silence. Be patient with yourself as it may take weeks to become comfortable with the stillness.

Keep in mind that prayer is sharing, asking or talking, while meditating is listening. In our daily lives we are bombarded with a myriad of sounds and sights: like TV, cell phones, and traffic. We have come to accept them as background noise. This meditation is a practice in listening to what is beneath that noise. There is a silence, a quiet that we rarely experience. It may take some time to hear or sense the answers you seek. This knowledge may come in words, flashes, pictures or simply a feeling.

Another benefit of this type of meditation is that it allows the mind and emotions to rest. The alpha and theta brain waves are also the optimum states for physical healing.

The first part of this meditation is *guided* and will help you attain the alpha state for internal self-awareness – beneath the interference of the ego – to be realized. It may be uncomfortable at first as old wounds and unresolved issues will be coming up for air. Take note of them then return your attention to the guided imagery.

To achieve the theta state through *unguided,* silent meditation, let go of all mental focus. This is the ultimate goal of meditation: to merge with your spiritual essence where all True Knowledge abides.

Deep Meditation
Instructions

☐ Sit or lie comfortably. Take several deep slow refreshing breaths. This will create a connection between your brain and your body, informing both that you are preparing for meditation. When you are ready to become still, imagine *one single object*, such as a candle flame or blade of grass, an ocean wave, a grain of sand, the sun or moon etc. You may also use a word, repeating it with your breath, words like peace, calm, bliss, safe, love, joy or Om.

☐ Close your eyes and let the word or object come to you now.

☐ As you focus on the word or object allow any mental pictures or thoughts to simply pass by like clouds. When you get distracted (this is normal), quietly bring your focus back to your object or word. Go into this without any expectation or effort as you are actively practicing *letting go* and just experiencing whatever comes to you.

☐ Then let go of the mental focus and surrender to silence as long as you can.

☐ You will come out of the meditation when you need to. You may only be able to stay in that space for a few minutes to begin with but with practice the time will increase.

☐ I recommend, at first, to set an alarm for 20 minutes, twice a day.

• Write down everything you've noticed after practicing any of these exercises for 30 days. This will help you to see the progress you've made. The rewards are worth the effort and you are worth the rewards.

As trite as this may sound, your entire life can change through a daily routine of meditation.

Chakra Imagery

Relaxation Imagery

Nature Imagery

Pain Reduction Imagery

Deep Meditation

Volume 2 in this series by Julie Bradshaw includes Shamanic Imageries for meeting your Spirit Guides, Animal Guides and developing intuition.

Hypnotherapy

I incorporate hypnotherapy, yet another healing tool like imageries or meditation, in counseling and healing sessions. Imageries are a form of hypnotherapy as the goal is the same: to quiet the conscious mind, create a mental and physical state of deep relaxation and make a positive life change.

What Hypnotherapy Is

Hypnotherapy is a learned skill and a process for assisting a client's desire towards achieving a specific goal such as: quitting smoking, weight control, relief from test anxiety, stress/pain reduction, retrieving repressed memories, behavior changes and past life regressions.

What Hypnotherapy is Not

Hypnosis is not being unconscious and at the mercy of the therapist's whims. You cannot be controlled or manipulated to quack like a duck at the count of three.

Imagery will induce the alpha or the theta brain wave state for relaxation. A hypnosis induction is geared towards maintaining the theta brain wave state in order to access the information within the subconscious or super-conscious for the purpose of achieving a goal.

The information recovered may answer questions such as, "What is holding me back from commitment?", "Where does this anxiety or anger stem from?", "What is the cause of my illness?", "Why am I not allowing myself to be happy?"

In a hypnotic state you are aware of your surroundings at all times and can speak, feel, sense and react as you wish at any time. You are simply in the deep state of theta brain waves. This is when you are most receptive to memories, suggestion and new concepts through affirmations.

As your conscious mind rests, your subconscious mind is more accessible. This state of being is remarkably efficient in its ability to re-script your habitual thought patterns and beliefs. The subconscious is where your ingrained ideas, principles and convictions lie. Often, they aren't even *yours*. They are your parents', friends' or teachers', but became part of your subconscious through repetition and it is through repetition that change of belief systems takes place.

One hypnotherapy session alone can't change an ingrained, deep-rooted belief. However, a session will inform you of that belief and then it will be your choice to accept it as yours or not. Put simply, you will become aware of the old tapes that have been running your life and can choose to begin creating new tapes. A series of sessions can help you do just that.

My experiences and those of my clients have found it to be an invaluable tool. I highly recommend that a healer take a reputable hypnotherapy course, become certified and continue studies in this field. Your expertise in hypnotherapy will aid in a healing practice exponentially.

Yoga Breathing Techniques

Yoga, Tai Chi and other meditative exercises are healthy for the body, mind and spirit. These breathing techniques add oxygen to the body and balances the energy meridians. Keep your tongue at the roof of your mouth to prevent hyperventilation in all breathing exercises. After each technique, sit quietly in meditation.

1. **Prana Yama – Nostril Breathing (10 times)**

- Place the middle finger of your right hand on your forehead. Put your thumb on your right nostril and your ring finger on your left nostril.

- Close your right nostril with your thumb and inhale through your left nostril deeply for a count of 8.

- Close both nostrils and hold your breath for a count of 4.

- Lift your thumb and exhale for a count of 8.

- Stay there and inhale for a count of 8 and hold your breath again for a count of 4. Close nostril.

- Release ring finger to exhale.

- Stay there and inhale for a count of 8 then hold for a count of 4. Close nostril.

- Release thumb to exhale.

- Repeat several times alternating sides.

  Benefits: Balances both hemispheres of the brain, clears sinuses, balances the nervous system, relieves the mind and has overall calming effect.

2. **Counting Breath – Long deep breathing (5 times or more)**

- Inhale to the count of 8 or more through the nose.

- Exhale to the count of 10 or more through the mouth as if through a straw. Empty the lungs completely and repeat the cycle.

  Benefits: Stress relief, stretching and strengthening the lungs for greater oxygen capacity.

3. **Heartbeat Breath - (7 times or more)**

- Place index and middle finger on one side of the Adam's apple to feel your pulse.

- Inhale for 8 heart beats.

- Hold for a count of 4 heartbeats.

- Exhale for 10 or more with each heartbeat.

  Benefits: Body awareness, lowering high blood pressure and developing patience for meditative practice.

4. Breath of Fire – (50 times each- 3 in succession)

- Inhale through the nostrils from your diaphragm (pushing your stomach out) and release the air quickly from your nostrils.

- Inhale again from your diaphragm and begin quick and fast in/out nostril breaths 50 times (Place a hand on your diaphragm to help focus and lower your shoulders.)

- Afterwards, relax with a long deep breathing.

  Benefits: Releases toxins, awakens the mind, energizes the body, improves circulation and concentration.

5. Korean Cleansing Breath - (100 times at 20 time increments)

- Inhale and pull stomach in tight.

- Exhale and push stomach out slowly 20 times (5 times a day).

- Afterwards, breathe a long deep breath.

  Benefits: helps with stomach problems, colitis, irritable bowl and hemorrhoids.

6. Standing Breath –

- Stand with feet shoulder width apart.

- Raise your arms above your head in prayer hand pose.

- Exhale 10 counts. Breathe in slowly for 8 counts then hold 4 counts while bending down from the waist at a 45° angle. This will force oxygen down to the lower part of the lungs.

  Benefits: Exercises the lower lung muscle for greater oxygen capacity. Extremely important for aging or illness.

Yoga Hand Mudras

Mudras (or hand positions) facilitate energy flow along the pathways (also called meridians or Nadis) of the body that induce specific states of body/mind consciousness.

Each finger correlates to a specific energy meridian. When one finger contacts another, a subtle energy circuit is created by the merging of these meridians.

Mudra Examples

Note: It is important to keep all fingers straight (except those touching others) to attain proper energy flow from the mudra being practiced.

1. **Namaste Mudra** (all meridian contact)

    How to: Place your palms together in prayer position.
    Benefits: Humility, respect for all, heart chakra, crown and third eye stimulation, balances both hemispheres of the brain.

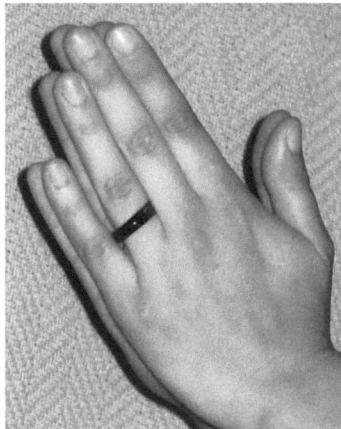

2. **Gyan Mudra**

    How to: Join the tips of the index finger and the thumb.
    Benefits: Induces meditation, wisdom, insights, vision, memory and joy.

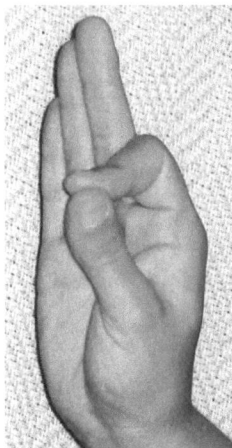

Apaan Mudra

How to: Join the tips of the thumbs to both the middle and ring fingertips.
Benefits: Stimulates the process of eliminating waste and toxins physically and mentally, clears head, eyes, ears and nose.

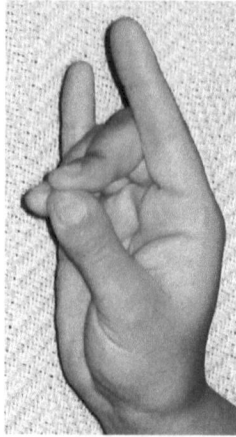

4. Prana Mudra

How to: Join the thumb to both the little and ring fingertips.
Benefits: Circulates and awakens life-force especially in the eyes.

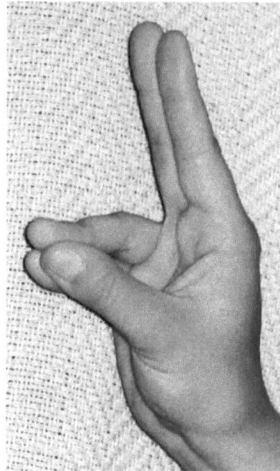

5. Surya Mudra

How to: Join the thumb to the ring fingertip.
Benefits: Overall strength, energy, vitality and joy.

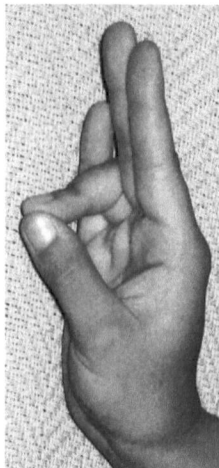

Varun Mudra

How to: Join the thumb to the little fingertip.
<u>*Benefits:*</u> Quality of the blood.

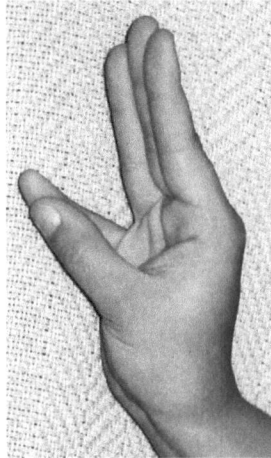

Sit quietly in meditation while using one mudra per meditation. The subtle nature of this energy through mudras is more effective after stretching, engaging in yoga, or any other physical activity.

Physical activities generate the energy and mudras serve to guide and direct that energy as each mudra is activated for a specific purpose or intent.

Hatha Yoga

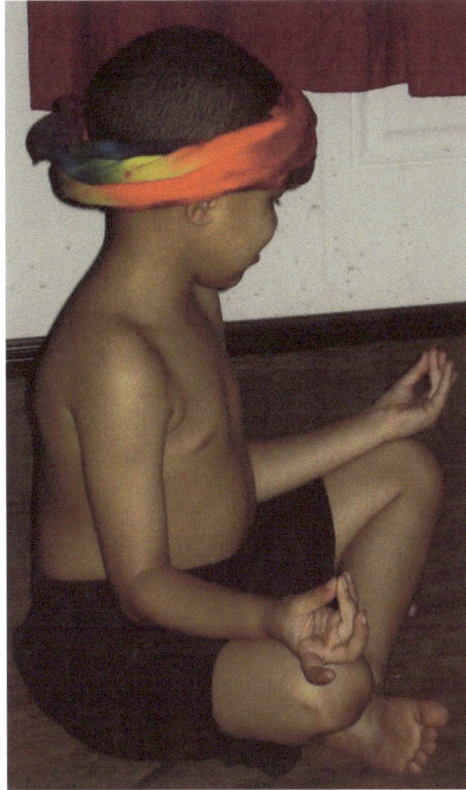

What is Hatha Yoga?

Like Tai Chi and Qi Gong of Chinese origin, yoga is another fascinating exercise consisting of precise movements, or poses, imbued with meaningful intentions.

As with the afore-mentioned practices, this exercise aims to elicit in the student a mindfulness of each move and each breath, resulting in a moving meditation. As the body is being stretched into a specific pose, the mind focuses solely on the body and directed breathing. By the end of the practice, the student is well prepared for a sitting meditation. A deeper meditation comes easily because of the relaxation of the body in conjunction with concentration of the mind.

In the sitting meditation, the Spirit (super-conscious) is exercised by chanting and eventually sitting in silence. Once the body, mind and Spirit are in union, the meditative experience can be an indescribable communion with all-ness (God, if you will).

This is not a vision or dialogue. It is a sense of True Peace. The beneficial results of this practice are numerous: Less stress, mental clarity, healthier body and spiritual insight. In essence, it improves the total human condition.

Yoga Evolves

Yoga is an established, possibly ancient practice. Archeological evidence of yoga poses were found illustrated on rock dating back to 3000 B.C., tracing its beginnings back to the Stone Age.

Shamanism is an ancient belief system whose central philosophy, evidenced in many cultures around the world, holds that if the individual is healthy and well balanced, in mind as well as body, so then the community will be balanced as well. Most Eastern cultures since, have maintained that belief.

Over five millennia, Yoga has evolved. Today, we can study its evolution, divided into four periods: The Vedic Period, the Pre-Classical Period, the Classical Period and the Post Classical period (or Modern Era).

Today, Yoga takes many different forms, from the more physically-oriented practices to the easy, restorative, meditative exercises. A student's individual needs and desires determine the choice of method.

The following photographs depict a few yoga poses. The instructions for each are based on the Hatha Yoga tradition, a slower, meditative practice. These poses open the primary chakras, the focal points of the body's "on" switches, to stimulate energy flow along the meridians and systems.

Yoga Poses

1. For each pose, follow these instructions while you hold the post for 1 to 2 minutes. Focus your eyes on one point in front of you (i.e. a speck on the wall, floor, ceiling).

2. Breathe in and out like ocean waves. On the exhale, let your entire body sink heavier into the pose but do not strain yourself. Continue to breathe and sink even deeper and heavier. Allow the weight of your body to do the stretching (not the will).

3. Very slowly and gracefully move to the next pose and repeat:
    *   Focus your eyes on one spot.
    *   Breathe and sink into the pose.

4. Repeat each pose 3 times before you move to the next pose.

5. Once you have finished all the poses, sit comfortably for your 20 to 45 minute meditation including a chant (page 215).

6. Chant as long as you wish.

7. Lastly, practice silence.

If you utilize this simple practice at least 3 times a week, you will experience dramatic changes in your overall attitude and behavior within a relatively short time. Yoga develops patience which creates a calming and more balanced lifestyle.

Yoga Poses

Mountain Pose

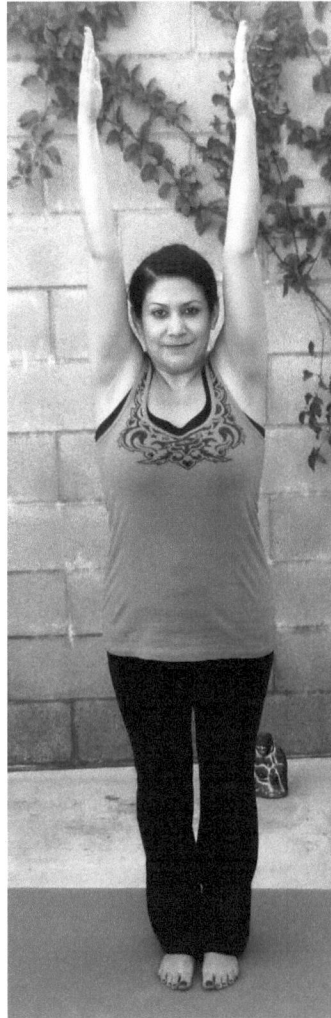

How to:

- Stand straight up with your feet planted about the width of your hips.

- Tuck in your bottom and tighten the muscles above your knees.

- Lift your chin up and out a little so it goes away from your shoulders. Now take a deep cleansing breath, filling your lungs to capacity.

- Lift your arms over your head with your hands open and facing each other.

- Soften and stretch from your shoulder joints. Fix your eyes on a distant point and hold this pose for a count of 10.

- Relax and let your arms drift back down to your sides (repeat 3 times).

<u>Benefits</u>**:** Helps to line up the spine, improves stance, distributes equilibrium to the mind and body.

Half Moon Pose

<table>
<tr><td align="center">Right</td><td align="center">Left</td></tr>
<tr><td>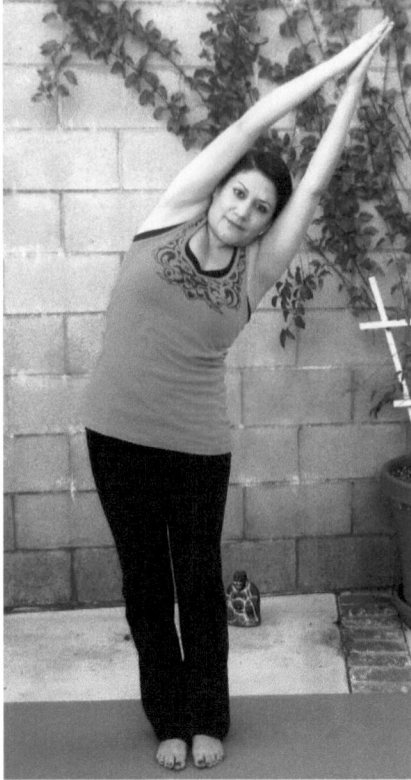</td><td>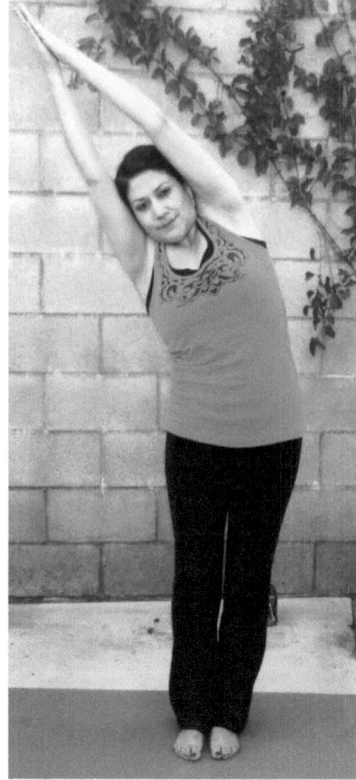</td></tr>
</table>

How to:

- Stand straight up feet a few inches apart.

- Lift both arms over your head with your palms facing.

- Squeeze the muscles just above the knee and gradually bend from your middle to the left side.

- Hold this position for a count of 5.

- Now come back to the starting position and lower your arms to your sides, relaxing your shoulders.

- Repeat the same steps for the right side.

- Do this pose 3 times for each side.

<u>*Benefits:*</u> Stretches and elongates the side muscles and strengthens the spine, arms and physical balance.

Yoga Mudra Pose

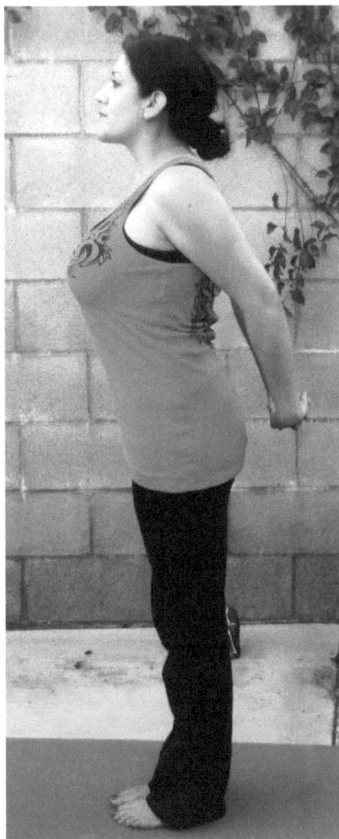
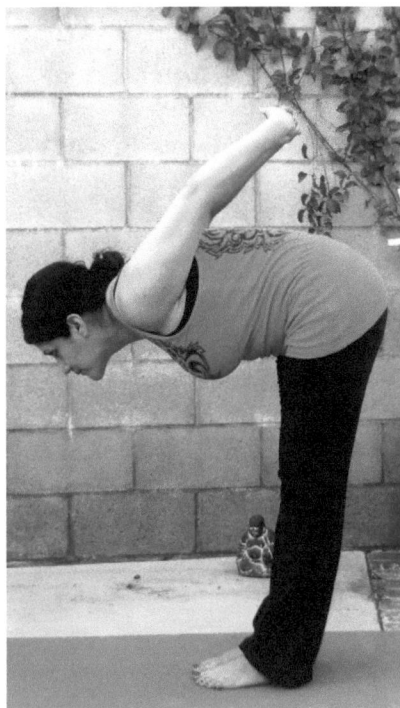

How to:

Picture 1

- Stand straight with your feet together a few inches apart.

- Reach behind you and interlace your fingers

- Keep your head looking straight forward.

Picture 2

- With your hands still behind your back, bow down from the hips, allowing your arms to come up behind you with the movement, your head facing your knees.

- Hold this pose for a count of 6.

- Breathing in, begin to straighten up little by little, allowing your arms to descend smoothly and raise your head slowly (repeat 3 times).

- Free your hands.

<u>Benefits:</u> Develops elasticity in the upper body including the waist, back, shoulders and neck, fortifies the legs, ankles and feet for better support, lengthens the spine, releases the hip area for greater mobility and enhances staying power and resilience.

Triangle Pose

Picture 1

Picture 2

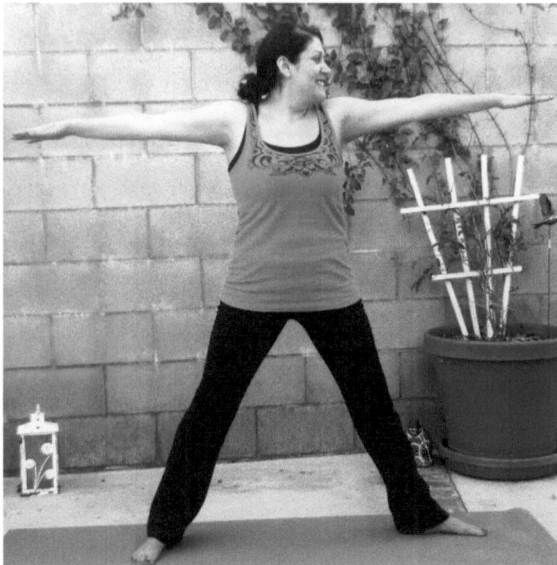

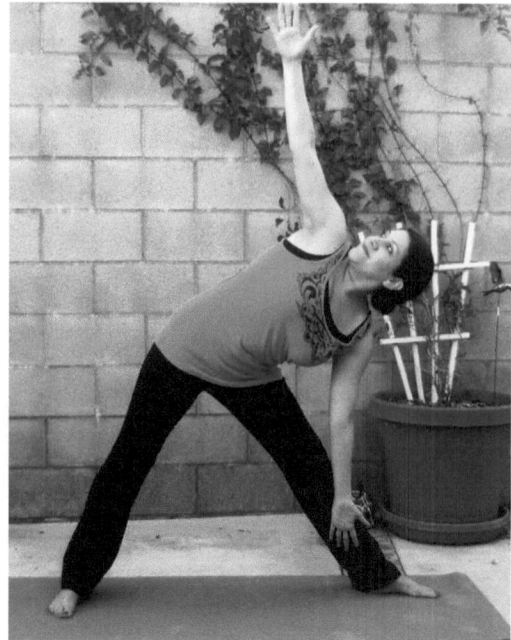

How to:

Picture 1

- Stand straight with your feet planted three feet apart.

- Now turn your right foot to point to the side.

- Move your left foot the opposite direction slightly, not as far as the right foot.

- Take a deep breath and raise your arms to shoulder height while moving your hips towards the front.

- Now shift your weight to the right side.

Picture 2

- Lean down from the waist on the right side, resting your right arm on your shin and reach up with your left towards the sky.

- Turn your head to look at your left thumb if you can without pulling too much. You want to feel the stretch but not cause injury.

- Hold this pose for 5-10 breaths

- Gently relax from this pose, give yourself a moment then repeat for the other side (repeat 3 times).

<u>Benefits:</u> Develops elasticity in the upper body including the waist, back, shoulders and neck, fortifies the legs, ankles and feet for better support, lengthens the spine, releases the hip area for greater mobility and enhances staying power and resilience.

Cat and Dog Stretch
Picture 1 (Cat Stretch)

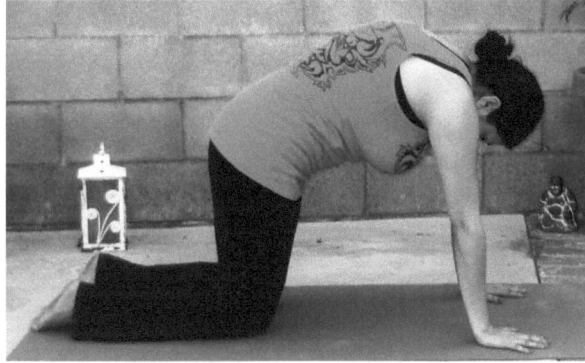

Picture 2 (Dog Stretch)

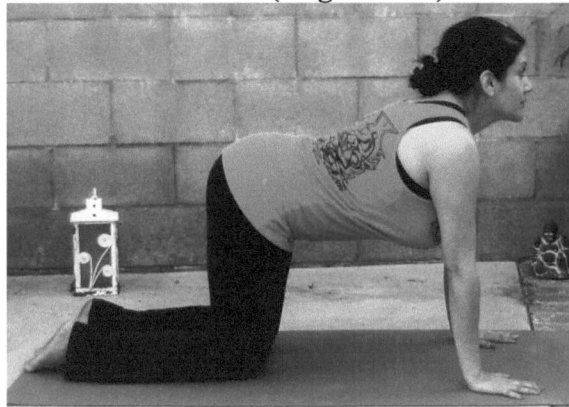

How to:

- Lower yourself down on your hands and knees like a table. Your knees should be aligned with your hips and your hands and arms with your shoulders.

- Keep your back flat and your head facing front.

Picture 1
- Release your breath and let your head and bottom tilt downward while curving your back upward naturally. Pull your bellybutton towards your spinal column and imagine a cat stretching, arching his back.

Picture 2
- Breathe in deeply and lift your head and bottom, letting your stomach release slowly towards the floor and look towards the sky. Imagine you are a friendly dog looking up for a treat.

- Switch between these two positions slowly several times. Take your time, breathing out for the cat (Picture 1) and in for the dog (Picture 2) positions.

Benefits: This stretch amplifies limberness along the entire back, increases circulation throughout the body and stretches the body all along the back, arms and neck.

Thunderbolt Pose

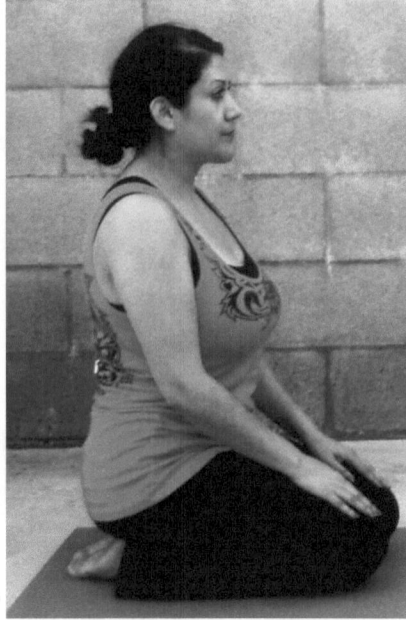

How to:

- Kneel down sitting back, with your legs about 6 inches apart with your feet extended out behind you.

- Face front with your arms set softly on your knees.

- You may close your eyes or focus on a point in front of you on the floor. Take a deep slow breath.

- Rest quietly in this pose as long as you need to.

<u>*Benefits:*</u> Supports a profound feeling of tranquility and peacefulness, enhances posture overall and bestows total relaxation.

Child Pose

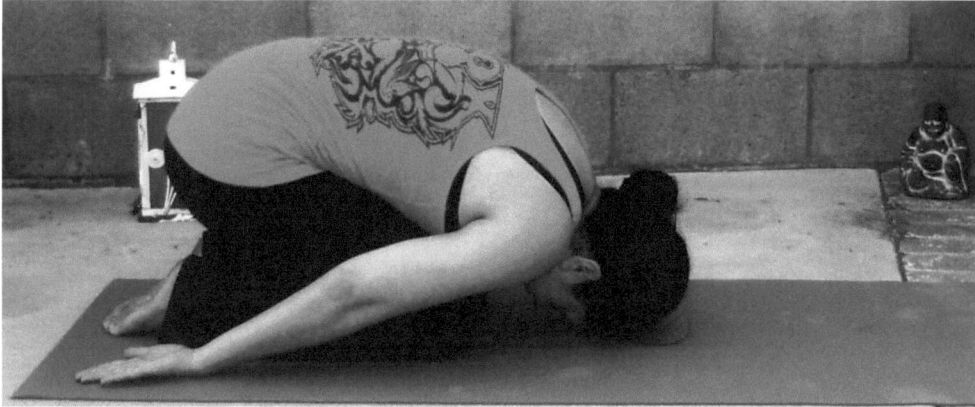

How to:

- Kneel down sitting back, with your legs about 6 inches apart with your feet extended out behind you.

- Lean down from the hips, moving forward and down, almost doubling your torso onto your legs with your forehead gently touching the floor.

- Set your arms next to your legs behind you, with your palms pointing towards the sky. An alternative move is to move your arms in front of you, past your head with your palms resting gently on the floor.

- Take slow deep breaths and unwind.

- Slowly lift first your arms, then your head and finally your torso and go back to the sitting position (repeat 3 times).

<u>Benefits:</u> Revitalizes the whole body, renews the back and spinal column, gently kneads the internal organs, supports a feeling of safety and growth.

Bent Knee Sitting Forward
Picture 1

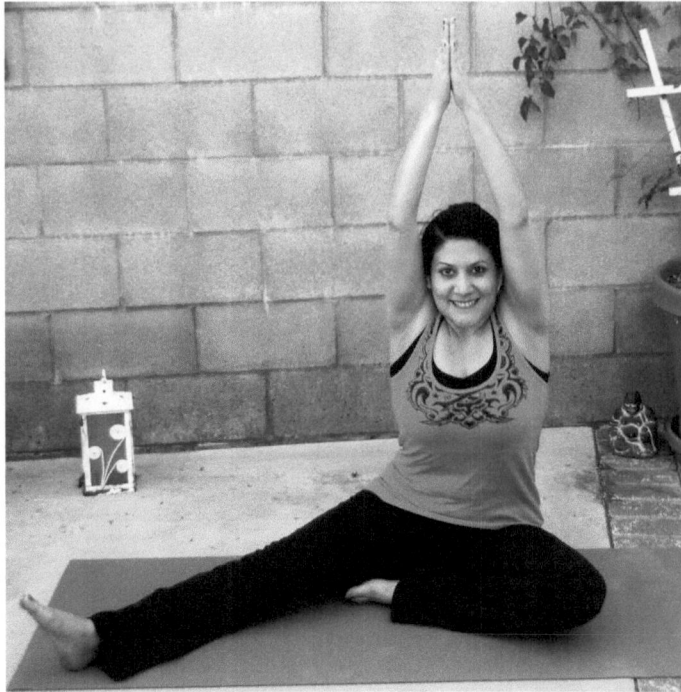

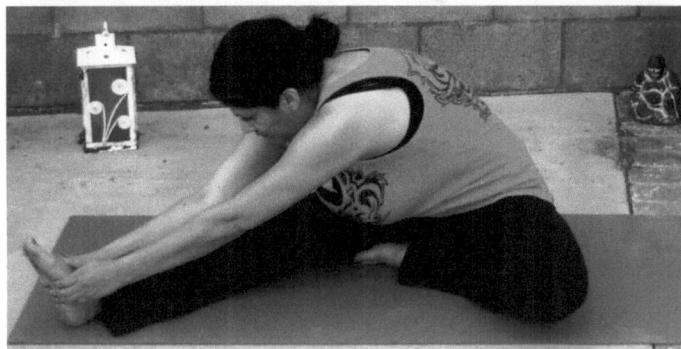

How to:

Picture 1
- Sit on your bottom, back straight and legs out in front of you. Bend one leg and let the bottom of that foot sit flat against the inside of the opposite leg.

- Take a deep breath and lift your arms up with your palms facing.

Picture 2
- Release the breath and lean down towards the extended leg. Stop when your back begins to curve out. Clasp the outstretched leg where you are able, at the knee, shin or foot, without pulling too hard. You may bend your leg slightly if that helps.

- Inhale into the position. As you exhale, fall deeply into the pose without effort.

- Duplicate for the other side by reversing the legs (repeat 3 times).

Benefits: Extends the hamstring muscles for greater flexibility, gently kneads the organs around the stomach, releases lower back pain and lends suppleness to the spine.

Reclining Spinal Twist

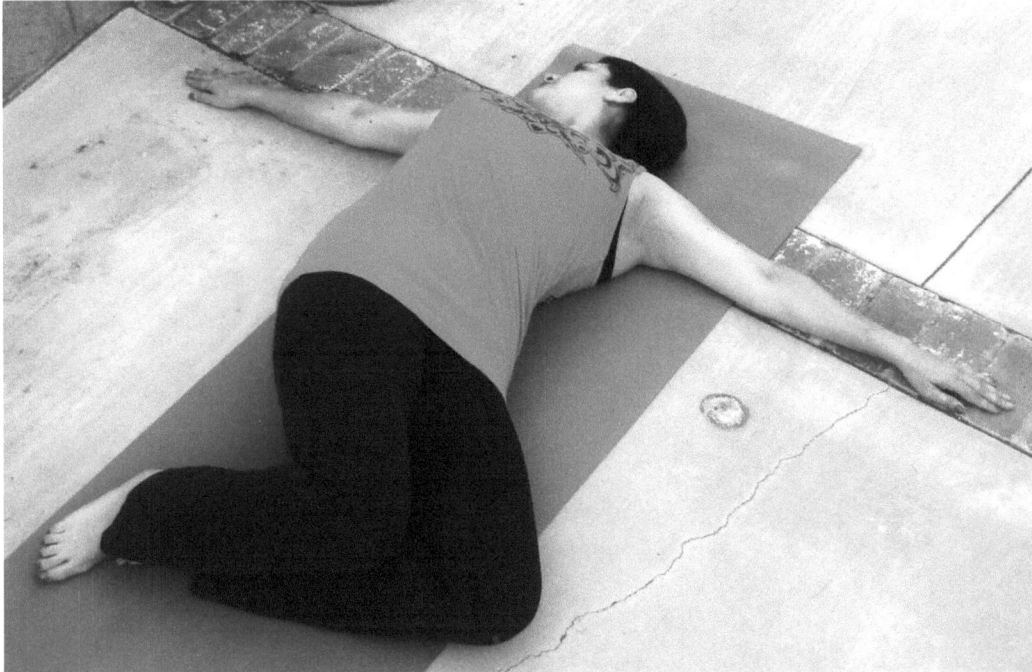

How to:

- Lie down flat on your back and pull your knees in so they are touching side by side.

- Stretch your arms out to your sides parallel with your shoulders so you look like the letter "T".

- Rotate only your legs and hips to the left side down to touch the floor. The right and left leg down to your feet should be stacked on top of one another.

- If your back curves, then move your knees closer to your chest.

- Twist your palms up towards the sky and move your arms into a "V" shape.

- Gently Turn your head to the right (opposite) direction of your knees.

- Permit your back to soften with each exhale and hold this pose for 1-2 minutes.

- Gradually move your legs and head back to center, leaving your arms in their current position.

- Reverse it for the other side (repeat 3 times).

Benefits: Relaxes the mind and balances the nervous system, alleviates headaches, cleans out the digestive tract and bowels and promotes equilibrium to the flow of Chi throughout the body.

Bound Angle (modified)
Picture 1

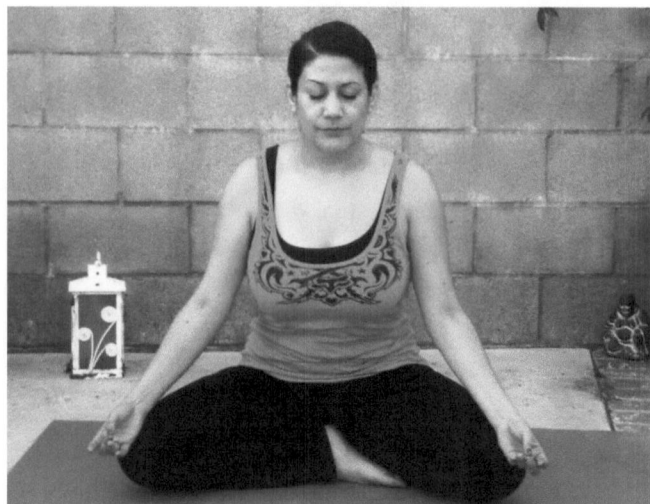

Picture 2

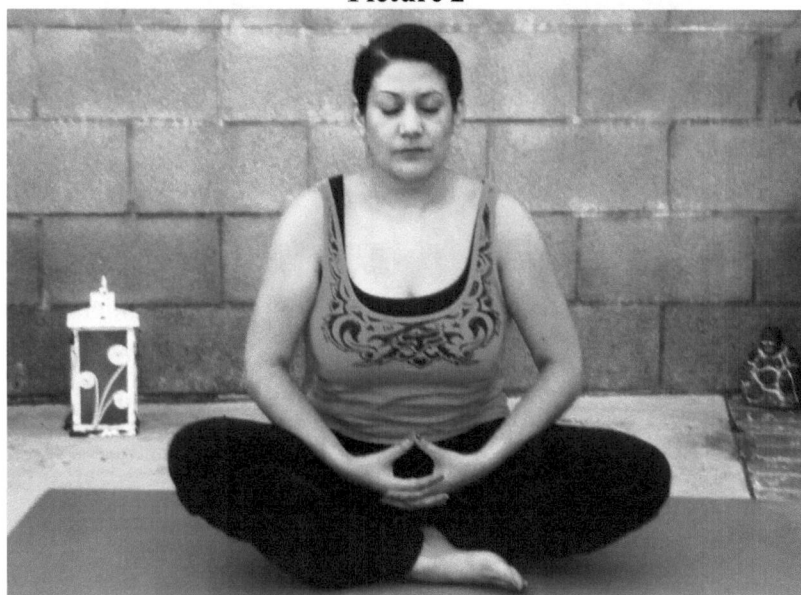

How to:
- Sit down on your bottom, your back straight. Put the bottoms of your feet together and lace your fingers around them (the picture 1, above shows a modified position with legs crossed; pictures 1 and 2 shows alternative hand placement).

- Rotate your shoulders down and forward away from your head.

- Now gradually drop your knees towards the ground without straining the movement.

- Take a deep breath while you do this. Permit the groin muscles to release more and more with each exhale.

Benefits: Helps to relax the groin muscles allowing more flexibility, aids posture, makes the tendons and muscles in the hips and knees more limber.

Test: Mind-Body Meditations
(For Certification)

Requirements:

Please answer each question on a *separate sheet(s) of paper*. For certification purposes include the following:

- **Your name**
- **Date you are completing this test**
- **Write/type out each question, then answer it.**

1) What is the difference between prayer and meditation?

2) What is the difference between imagery and meditation?

3) What are the benefits of both?

4) What is your favorite imagery and meditation?

5) What was your personal experience?

6) Explain the 4 brain wave states.

7) Which one of the brain wave states are you eliciting for your client?

8) Why is yoga breathing beneficial?

9) Which of the yoga breathing techniques do you like most and why?

Chapter 5

Preparation for Healers

"Faith is a knowledge within the heart,
beyond the reach of proof."
Kahilil Gibran

Preparation for Healers: An Introduction

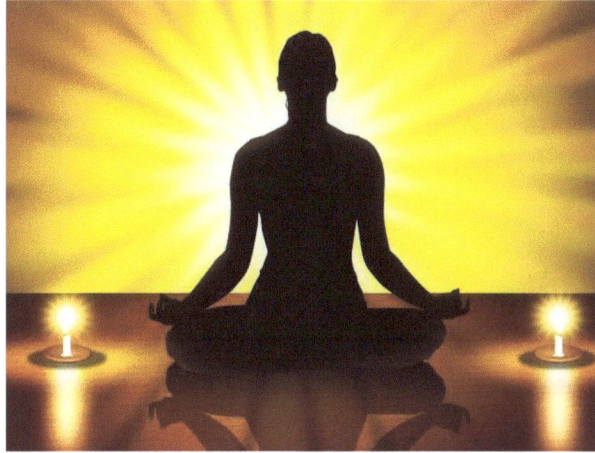

So far you have learned about yourself, the nature of energy, why we meditate, Chakras and Chi. The next step is preparing yourself to facilitate a healing.

It may seem as if there is a lot of information to take in, a lot of work to do before you get to the actual goal of performing a healing. There is. Directing and channeling energy to assist in healing another human being is not to be taken lightly.

Anything worthwhile takes time, effort and commitment to achieve. This is especially true in the healing arts. You are nurturing a connection with Spirit to help heal others and, by proxy, yourself. Any human-to-human relationship takes time to grow. Trust, respect and compassion are all earned within that relationship over time. The relationship with Spirit is no different. Be patient, you've come a long way.

The following chapters reveal several different healing techniques. If you refer back to the introduction of the book, you'll see we mentioned the progression of the chapters, one building on the other. Now you will begin to see (if you haven't already) how the connections between the body, mind, energy and spirit are all interwoven like a fine tapestry.

Spiritual Ups and Downs

There may be times when you have trouble connecting to your Divine Source. Do not be discouraged. It happens to the best of us. Why does even the Dalai Lama continue to meditate?

We are all reaching for spiritual fulfillment, however, we are also having a human experience at the same time. One of Julie's teachers in Ireland, Martin, says "It would be nice and wonderful to stay in this sacred space all the time. But you still have to do the laundry." And he's so right. We have to brush our teeth, eat, sleep, drive, work, take care of a family and if we're able to carve out time for spiritual practice, then great! For those very reasons, many of us do not have the luxury of focusing solely on spiritual disciplines. We have to take care of regular life's business. Again, here is where we try to find a balance between the two. Once we find it, it's like trying to hold a passing cloud in your hands. It will slip and drift between your fingers. The boss will call and say you need to stay overtime to finish a project. "But", you cry, "I was going to meditate tonight!" Understand that this, too, is part of the spiritual practice. These are the challenges on which character is built. How you handle each instance is what will help you to learn and grow as a healer and as a human *being*.

There is an old Zen saying: Before enlightenment- Chop wood, carry water. After enlightenment- Chop wood, carry water.

Life is like a wave, the tides ebb and flow on a regular basis. If you are at a place in your practice where you are connected on a regular basis then your spiritual cup is "full". Sometimes it must be emptied before it can be filled again. When you hit those walls, take them as a spiritual housecleaning, not a failure. You are preparing to receive even more gifts from Spirit.

As you study the next chapters, you will find that some techniques are quite easy, while others take more effort. As you begin to work with others in healing, keep a journal of your experiences, ideas and revelations. Over the course of time, you will be amazed at and proud of your development.

Moving forward

First, we will cover Basic Organs of the Body and the Endocrine System. It's important to know the locations of organs and glands when scanning for anomalies and using a localized healing modality.

The Aromatherapy, Muscle Testing, Channeling and Healing Procedures that follow are equally as important in the preparation to perform a healing.

Endocrine System

7th Chakra - Pineal Gland:
The Pineal Gland is also called the "Crown". It produces melatonin which affects wake/sleep patterns and seasonal functions. The production of melatonin by the pineal gland is stimulated by darkness and inhibited by light. It resembles a tiny pinecone, about the size of a grain of rice and historically was referred to as the "seat of the soul".

6th Chakra - Pituitary Gland:
About the size of a pea, the Pituitary Gland is also called the "master gland" or "Third Eye". It helps to control the bodily processes of growth, blood pressure, child birth (labor), sex organs (male/female), thyroid gland, the conversion of food into energy and balancing water (via re-absorption by the kidneys).

5th Chakra - Thyroid Gland:
The Thyroid Gland resembles a butterfly and is located at the throat. It is mainly responsible for turning food into energy, cell growth and regulation of other hormones in the body.

4th Chakra – Thymus Gland:
Located behind the sternum, its name comes from the Greek word 'thumos', meaning heart, soul, desire, life. It's main function is based in the immune system by producing T-cells.

3rd Chakra – Pancreas Gland:
The pancreas is located in the center of the kidneys, slightly lower than the adrenal gland. It does double duty as a regulator of glucose in the body (glucagon and insulin –raising and lowering glucose) as well as sending digestive enzymes into the small intestine to further break down carbohydrates and proteins. These two actions work independently of each other, as if they were separate.

2nd Gonads (Male- testes & Female- ovaries):
Located in the lower abdomen, they produce the hormones estrogen/progesterone in females and testosterone in males and also are responsible for the production of eggs and sperm.

1st Chakra – Adrenal Glands:
The Adrenals are situated on top of the kidneys, one on each side. They produce the hormones cortisol (increases blood sugar, metabolizing carbohydrates/proteins and suppressing the immune system-muting the white blood cells), aldosterone (increases blood volume/pressure and water retention – aiding the kidneys) and androgens (male sexual development aka testosterone). They are also responsible for the 'flight or fight' response in the body, sourced by the Root Chakra.

Note: Ancient people discovered these precise locations by feeling the loci of energy and somehow recognize them as essential focus' for health. Today we know these are the locations of the endocrine system, the foundation of the immune system.

Endocrine System
Female & Male

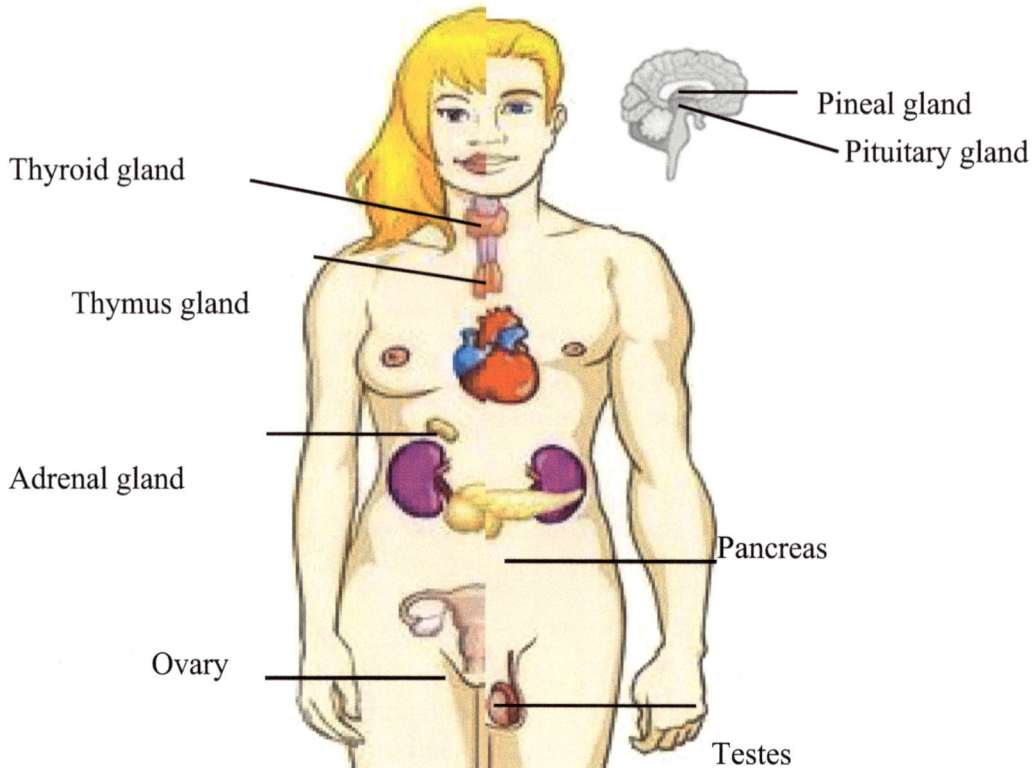

Pineal gland

Pituitary gland

Thyroid gland

Thymus gland

Adrenal gland

Pancreas

Ovary

Testes

Basic Anatomy

Aside from the general healing formats or blueprints taught in this manual, concentrating on healing specific organ issues of a client is important.

The healing formats are a launching pad. Throughout the healing, you can incorporate acupressure points, color, stones, sounds, etc. and spend time on an affected or imbalanced organ and gland.

Knowing the locations and functions of the organs is, of course, required. The more you educate yourself, the better you are as a healer. On the next page is a list of some of the major organs. It is by no means a complete list, as the human body is remarkably complex. With a simple search online or at your local book store, you can find several reference materials on organs and their functions. Gray's Anatomy Coloring Book is an excellent source for the detailed workings of the organs and other systems.

Bladder: This is the organ that stores urine (liquid waste) before expelling it from our bodies.

Brain: The brain is the control center of the body. It stores all experiences and is the source of thought, moods and emotions.

Endocrine System (Immune System): The endocrine system is a collection of glands that secrete hormones. The hormones pass through the blood to each organ, resulting in a chemical change in the body. It is the foundation of the immune system.

Gall Bladder: A sack where bile secreted by the liver is stored until needed by the body for digestion.

Heart: Maintains the flow of blood through the entire circulatory system to supply oxygen to the body.

Kidneys: A pair of organs which maintain proper water/electrolyte balance and filter the blood of metabolic wastes which are later excreted as urine.

Large Intestines: Extract moisture from food residues which are later excreted as feces.

Liver: Secretes bile and metabolizes carbohydrates, fats and proteins. This organ works very hard to keep all the impurities filtered out of our bodies from food, water and air.

Lungs: Remove carbon dioxide from the blood and provide it with oxygen.

Nervous System: Cells, tissues and organs that regulate the body's responses to internal and external stimuli. It consists of the brain, spinal cord, nerves and ganglia (a mass of nerve tissue existing outside of the central nervous system).

Nose: The part of the human face that contains nostrils which are lined with sensory nerves. It is the organ of smell and forms the beginning of the respiratory tract. Smell has the greatest influence of the 5 senses.

Pancreas: Lies behind the stomach and secretes pancreatic juice, insulin, glucagon and somatostatin which helps regulate the growth hormone in the body.

Small Intestines: The upper portion of the bowel in which most digestion occurs.

Spinal Cord: Nerve tissue that extends down through the spinal column and from which the spinal nerves branch off to various parts of the body.

Stomach: A principal organ of digestion.

Note: The stomach and intestines, (the storage tanks) need to maintain their PH balance. The health of these organ chakras is essential for longevity. Probiotics through foods like yogurt or through supplements are important to add to your diet.

Major Organs
Front View

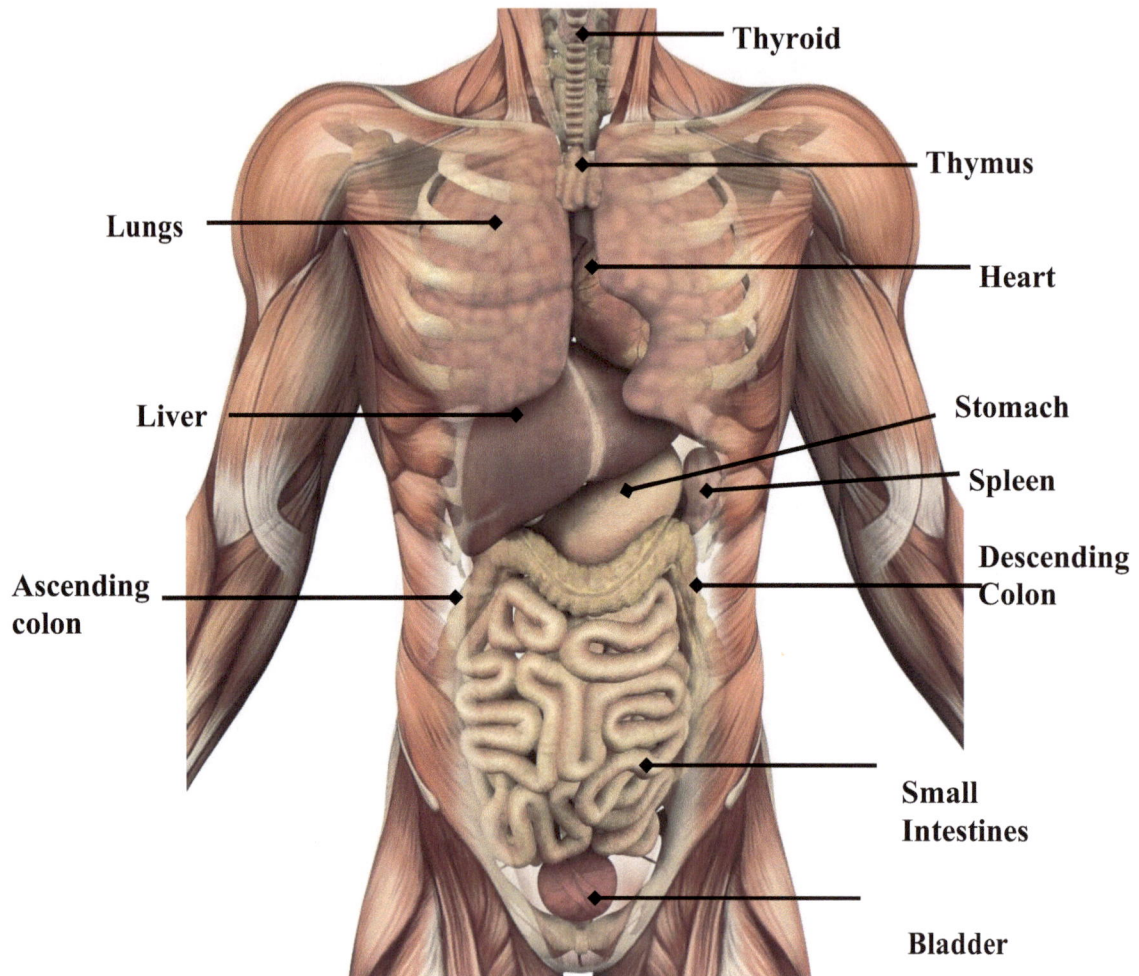

Thyroid

Thymus

Lungs

Heart

Liver

Stomach

Spleen

Ascending
colon

Descending
Colon

Small
Intestines

Bladder

Major Organs
Back View

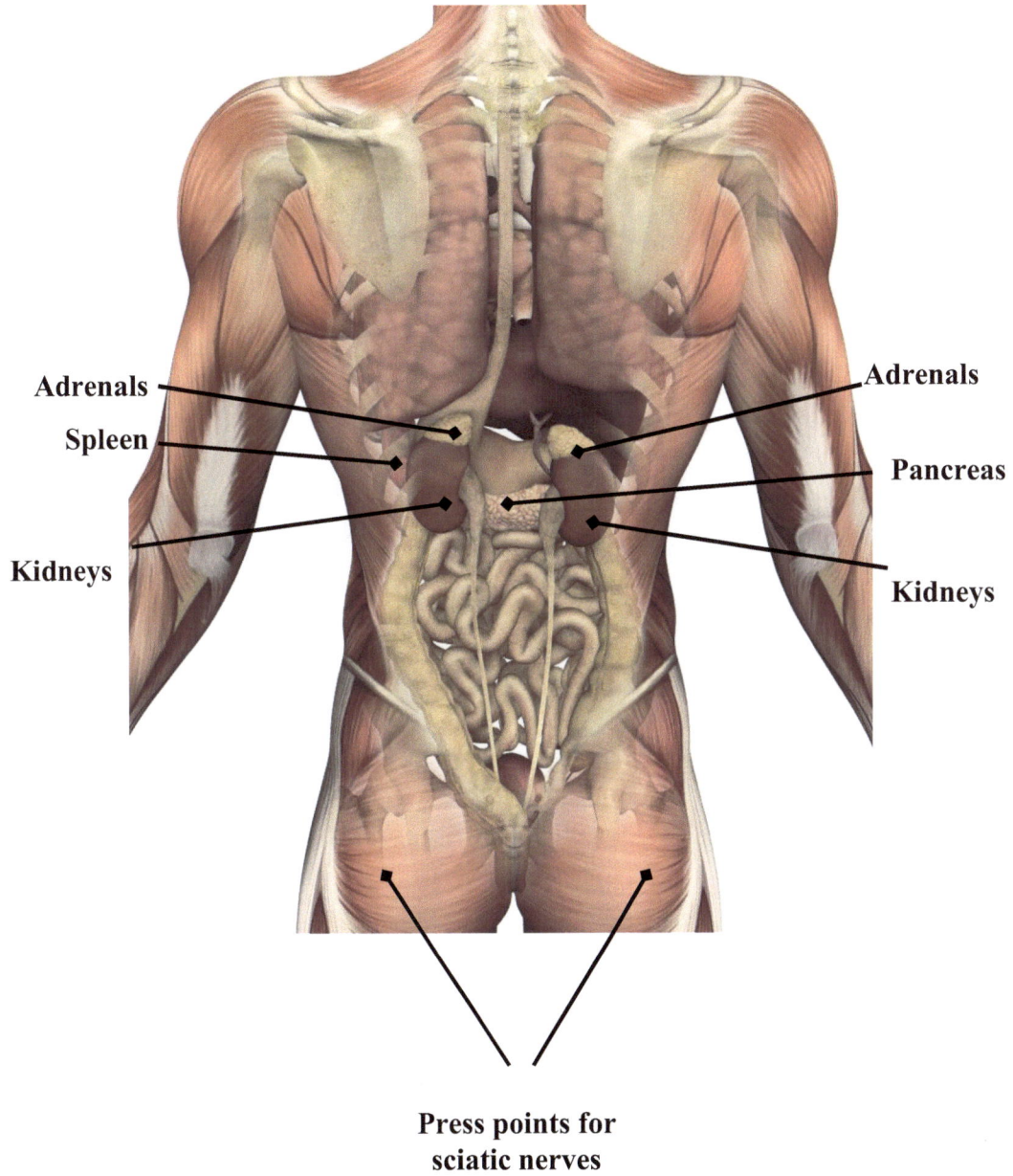

Adrenals

Adrenals

Spleen

Pancreas

Kidneys

Kidneys

Press points for
sciatic nerves

Skeletal Locations
Back View

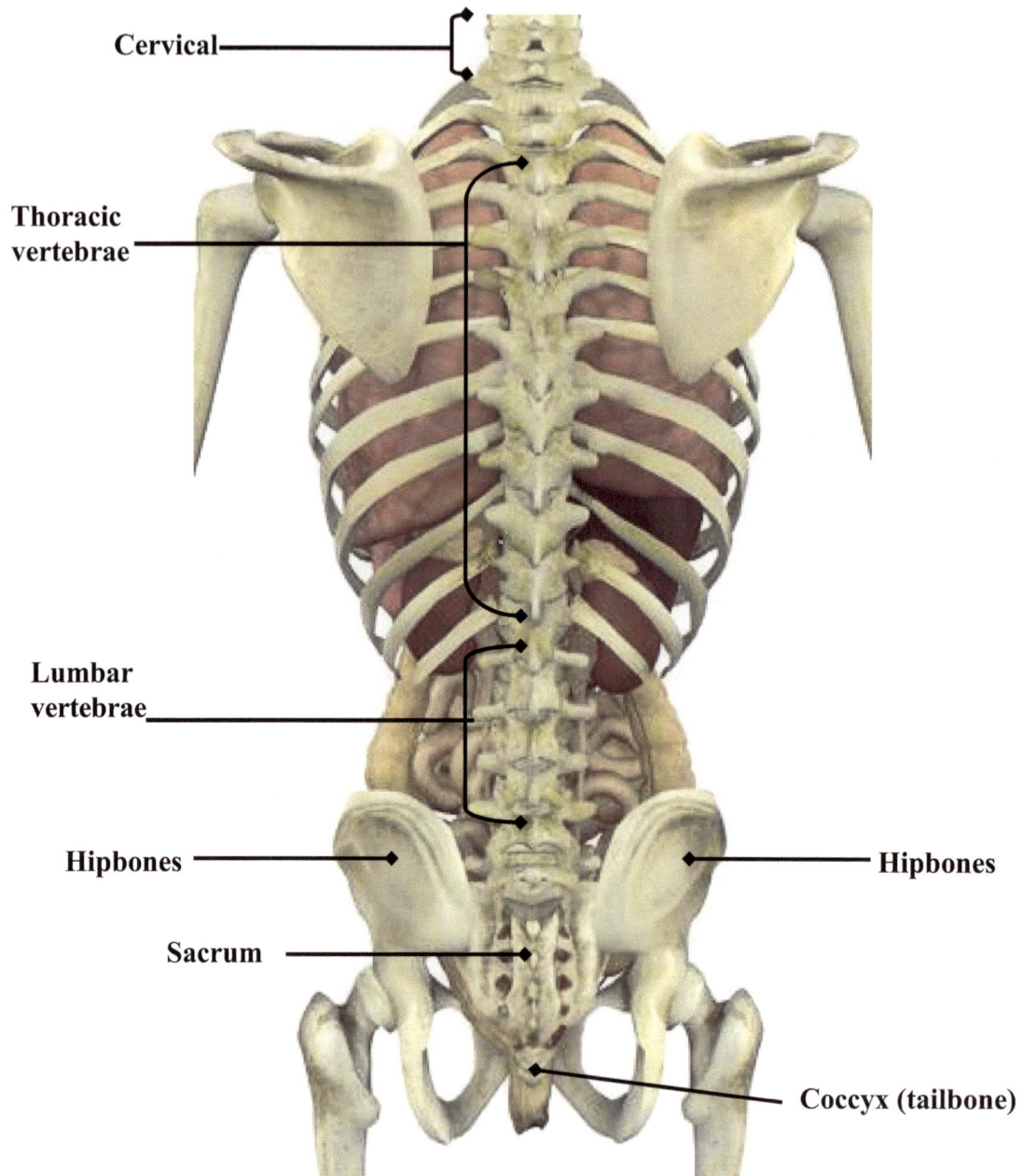

Cervical

Thoracic
vertebrae

Lumbar
vertebrae

Hipbones

Sacrum

Hipbones

Coccyx (tailbone)

Male & Female Reproductive Organs

These organs are located in the lower abdomen slightly below and in front of the small intestines.

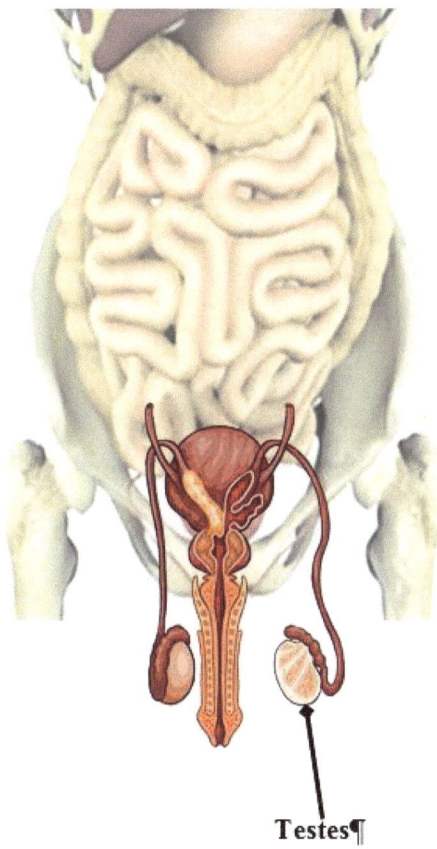

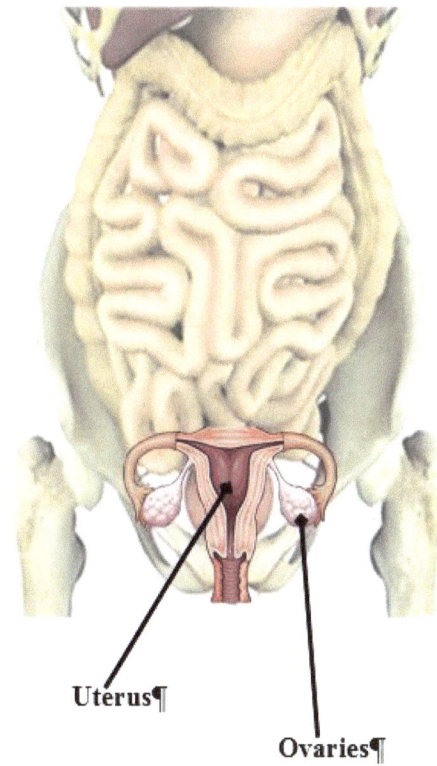

Uterus¶

Ovaries¶

Testes¶

Aromatherapy

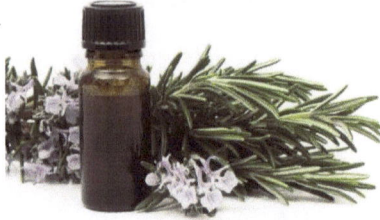

Ah, the smell of roses; Grandma's apple pie baking in the oven; your father's aftershave. All these scents are frequently associated with memories and/or emotions. The sense of smell is powerful and can trigger a happy memory or warn us of danger, as in the case of fire. That is why aromatherapy is an excellent tool to add to your healing "toolbox". It helps your client to associate the aroma with healing, with feeling whole, vibrant and healthy.

If your desire is to learn how to blend oils for remedies, you must either take courses to become an aromatherapist or else *strictly* follow recipes from credible sources. Do not "play" with essential oils. Aromatherapy is often mistaken as being solely a perfume or scent. It is, rather, the use of essential oils extracted from plants to promote healing processes for physical or psychological disorders. The medicinal properties of these plants have powerful qualities and, if blended properly, may be very beneficial to your client and will do no harm.

However, some oils when taken internally can be harmful to the liver, as the liver is the organ primarily responsible for processing and eliminating unwanted substances and chemicals from the body, therefore excesses of even beneficial substances can accumulate and cause damage.

Aromatherapy is just another healing tool. Take care to treat it as you would any tool out of your garage. Much like a hammer, it can repair something or it can damage it.

Also note, there are several species of flora that are poisonous. Generally, essential oils of these plants are not sold to the public, therefore, it is imperative that you *do your research*. For instance, Cinnamon is especially irritating to most skin types but may be used in aromatherapy if applied to a tissue rather than the hands.

There are a number of resources via the Internet from which you can learn about essential oils and their history. India, China, Rome, Egypt, England, Greece and many locations from the Biblical era all have a history utilizing these oils.

Because Mother Earth provides us with all we need, the "blood" of plant life offers a wealth of life-supporting aides. Essential oils carry properties that render them anti-inflammatory, antiviral, antibacterial, antifungal, or antiseptic. They also can relieve anxiety, depression, insomnia and digestive problems, as well as stimulate the nervous system, lower high blood pressure, improve mental acuity and much more.

On a physiological level, essential oils directly impact the hormonal system, which in turn directly affects the immune system, strengthening and balancing it.

Most aromatherapy blends (and spices) are non-toxic and are therefore a great supplement to use for many conditions. For example, I use Turmeric with CBD oil for bursitis.

If you choose to use aromatherapy in your healing practice, you must learn how to use the oils properly. Many pure essential oils will burn the skin if not mixed with base oil. Some essential oils, however, can be used undiluted as a mouthwash or for cooking.

There are many uses for pure essential oils such as compresses, in massage therapy or as air fresheners. They can be applied topically or more frequently inhaled using burners, vaporizers or steam, as well as inhaling from a tissue or straight from the palms of the hands. You can also apply several drops of pure essential oils, such as orange or peppermint, on a piece of cloth and place it in a dryer load. Your clothes will carry these subtle scents throughout your day.

Take the time to become well-educated in mixing oils so you can customize blends for your clients. I love the skill and art of aromatherapy and as in any art, I find that the more I learn, the more there is to learn.

I suggest buying or making three blends to start off with as a healer: *Relaxation, Sacred* and *Energizing*. Below are three simple recipes to make on your own.

What you will need
Pure essential oils.
Almond oil, used as a base.
Glass bottles with screw on lids.

There are many selections of base oils including: olive oil, primrose, apricot, calendula and comfrey. All have different properties. Sweet almond oil is a good starting point because it has no dominant scent of its own and therefore won't hinder the essential oil's scent, making it more evident.

Recipes

The Proper Ratios
First, you'll need to know the correct amount of base oil for the size of bottle you're blending. See table below.

Next, you will be adding the essential oils to the base oil for your blend. Refer to this table for amounts and sizes of bottles to use.

Base Oil Amount	=	Bottle Size
1 Teaspoon	=	5ml
2 Teaspoon	=	10ml
3 Teaspoon	=	15ml

Essential Oil Amount to be added to base oil	=	Bottle Size
2 - 5 drops	=	1 Teaspoon base oil / or 5ml bottle
4 - 10 drops	=	2 Teaspoon base oil / or 10 ml bottle
6 - 15 drops	=	3 Teaspoon base oil / or 15ml bottle

Basic Aroma Recipes for Healing

For each aroma recipe listed, begin with a **5ml bottle and add 1 teaspoon of your chosen base oil** from the table on the previous page. Then add the essential oils from one of the chosen recipes below:

Note: Each recipe will yield one- 5 ml blend

Relaxation
3 drops Ylang Ylang
1 drop Lavender
1 drop Bergamot

Sacred (also relaxing)
2 drops Sandalwood
2 drops Frankincense
1 drop Clary Sage

Energy
1 drop Peppermint
2 drops Rosemary
2 drops Orange

How to use aromatherapy in a healing

At the beginning of a healing, place a couple of drops of *Relaxation* or *Sacred* blend (according to the client's scent preference) on the client's palm and have them rub their palms together and breathe it in 5 times. This will trigger the client's olfactory sense (sense of smell) and create an association between the scent and the healing effects they are about to receive. Afterwards, continue with the healing.

Additionally, I will often use the same blends on my own palms before a healing to scan the client's auric field.

After the healing, do the same with the energy blend. This will help the client feel refreshed, invigorated and ready to face the world.

More is *not* better. This is quite enough in a one hour session. In fact, using more than 2 different blends a day is not recommended. If a certain aroma is used too much or too often, the result may be the exact opposite of that blend. For example: Breathing in the Energy blend for too long may cause drowsiness or breathing in Lavender too long may cause agitation.

Keep in mind that some people have allergies to oils, such as peppermint or tea tree. Make sure to discuss with your client what allergies they may have to determine which scents may or may not be right for them. Aromatherapy is also an excellent replacement for incense if you have clients with lung or breathing problems.

Aromatherapy Chakra Blends

As with the Basic healing blends, these recipes will also yield one-5 ml each.
Use 1 tsp base oil into a 5 ml bottle then add the following oils for the corresponding Chakra point you wish to concentrate on to balance in the healing.

Crown Chakra
2 drops Lavender or Rose
3 drops Frankincense

Brow Chakra
2 drops Lavender or Chamomile
2 drops Clary Sage
1 drop Sandalwood

Throat Chakra
1 drop Peppermint
1 drop Spruce
1 drop Thyme

Heart Chakra
1 drop Lime
1 drop Eucalyptus
1 drop Ylang Ylang
1 drop Camphor or Cedar

Solar Plexus Chakra
1 drop Juniper
2 drops Ginger
1 drop Chamomile
1 drop Jasmine or Lemon

Spleen (2nd) Chakra
1 drop Geranium
2 drops Sandalwood
2 drops Patchouli

Root Chakra
1 drop Clove
1 drop Pine
1 drop Patchouli
2 drops Sage

Essential Oil Properties

- ◆ **Ylang Ylang** – *Stress, high blood pressure, anxiety*

- ◆ **Lavender** – *Calming, antiseptic, eczema, scars*

- ◆ **Bergamot** – *Depression, anxiety, digestion*

- ◆ **Sandalwood** – *Meditation, skin problems, aphrodisiac*

- ◆ **Frankincense** – *meditation, lungs, anti-inflammatory*

- ◆ **Myrrh** – *Skin problems, lungs, digestion*

- ◆ **Peppermint** – *Digestion, motion sickness, muscle pain, colds*

- ◆ **Rosemary** – *Circulation, fatigue, concentration, headaches, sprains*

- ◆ **Orange** – *Constipation, tiredness, relaxation, uplifting*

These are just a few examples of oils and their healing properties. As you research, you will find an abundance of information on these and numerous other essential oils. All essential oils are derived from plants and our planet is home to hundreds of thousands of species.

Optional Base Oils

- ◆ **Sweet Almond Oil** – *Unscented, all skin conditions, soothing*

- ◆ **Evening Primrose** – *Skin problems, PMS/Menopause, heart disease*

- ◆ **Olive oil** – *Rheumatic conditions, inflamed skin, aches*

- ◆ **Calendula** – *Anti-inflammatory, skin problems, stretch marks*

- ◆ **Comfrey** – *Scars, arthritis, pain, broken bones, burns*

- ◆ **Jojoba** – *Anti-inflammatory, dry skin, acne, skin problems*

- ◆ **St. John's Wort** – *Nerve pain, backache, shingles, antiseptic*

Volume 2 of the Series includes healing herb and spice recipes for teas and sachets.

Muscle Testing
For Aromas, Supplements or Foods

    With aromatherapy blends, you will find several oils that will elicit relaxation, energy and other blends that may aid in relieving high blood pressure, insomnia or other conditions.

    How do you choose which oils to use for a client? Muscle testing is one way to do this.

    For example, lavender and chamomile both have relaxation effects, however, they also have different unique properties as well. By muscle testing, you can determine which essential oil will be most effective for your client.

How to Muscle Test

1. Stand facing your client and have them smell and breathe in one aroma 3 times.
2. Then have them hold the bottle of that aroma in their left (receiving) hand.
3. Now, have them hold their right arm out to their side at shoulder height.

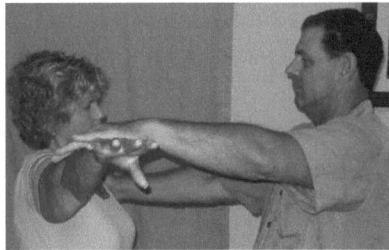

4. Place your right hand on their left shoulder and your left hand on their right wrist.
5. Tell them to resist as you push their arm down towards the floor.

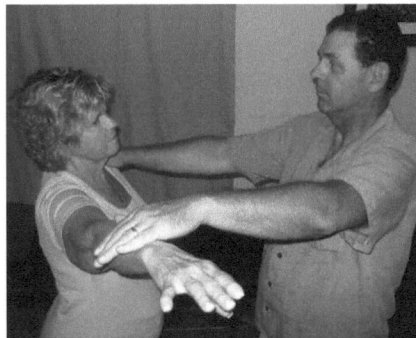

6. If their arm barely moves, that means the oil is strengthening for them and consequently is a healthy choice.

7. If their arm drops downward, then the opposite is true. The oil is weaker and not the best choice for this client at this time.

    Test each oil this way until you narrow them down to the 3-5 best choices and there's your aromatherapy blend, custom-made for your client.

    You can utilize this procedure with foods, vitamins, mineral supplements and anything else that applies. It is not a good idea, however, to ignore instructions for any over-the-counter medications or supplements you are considering. This is simply another tool and guide. Use common sense and follow the labels.

What is Channeling?

Many people hear the word "channeling" and respond immediately with apprehension or trepidation. "What is *that*? Some kind of ghost thing?" No, it isn't. In fact, we all channel unconsciously on a daily basis. Inspirations, insights, music, poetry and even mathematics are the creativity we channel into ourselves. Where does the realm of ideas originate from? Where did Einstein draw his relativity theory from? How did Edison come up with the vision of light bulbs? These are original ideas, original concepts, a first of their kind.

Some ideas surfaced from the subconscious. This is not necessarily channeling. For example: out of 50 songs I wrote, maybe three were really good. One in particular was downright great. When my brother heard it, he really enjoyed it and then added, "It sounds a little familiar". Over the next few weeks, my long-term memory files opened up. "Oh yeah", I thought, "half of that melody came from that Ella Fitzgerald song I heard 20 years ago, dang it". I still love my variation of that song as I laugh over my increasingly granny bad memory. This song came from my *sub*conscious to my *conscious*.

But then there are truly original ideas that come from our *super*-conscious. Our brain is not our mind. Our brain is the *receptacle of our consciousness* and the *interpreter of our experiences.*

I had a client who had frequent vivid dreams and benefited from dream analysis. She had one such dream when she asked, "Why is Mickey Mouse pulling me out of the quicksand?" (Interpreting dreams is hardly complex, by the way, once you know the right questions to ask yourself.) After we talked, she was able to identify the quicksand as her fears of "going under". She was overwhelmed by the burdens of her present life. She loved Disneyland with a passion and hadn't been able to go for quite a while. She, with no prompting from me, realized that Mickey Mouse was telling her to get out of the mire and have some fun, get refreshed, laugh, lighten up.

Our brain interprets and deciphers information that comes from all emotions and experiences. This vibrational information is interpreted by the brain, often associating it with pictures, colors and sounds by a cognitive/conscious understanding. Most often, dreams are pictorial associations originating from the subconscious.

Sometimes, however, dreams are the result of a gateway to and from the super-conscious. Our brain is an organ, sending and receiving information much like a computer. Original thoughts, however, come from an outer source- the creator of the brain/computer. There are the subconscious, conscious and super-conscious. The super-conscious is the greater mind outside of your three dimensional existence.

Some call it the "higher self" or the soul. Meta-physics literally means "beyond and above the physical". Our higher mind is still a mystery but may be experienced in meditation, dreams and unexplained "knowings" ("It just popped into my head one day"). Our expanded mind, when freed from the body and brain, unites with the vibrational information of the universe, the God/Higher Power; the other dimensions of existence.

After meditations, dreams and near-death experiences, many people have adamantly insisted that the experiences they've had were real.

There is no question or doubt in their minds. The sense of wholeness with all life's creations, the visits with loved ones on the other side, the greater understanding of existence and the knowledge otherwise never considered by them before this experience, are all very real.

The collective consciousness of man resides, as well, in the super-conscious. We call it telepathy. And so, when we are channeling for the purpose of healing, we are channeling energy and information from the super-conscious, the greater mind united with the universe/God; innate knowledge of vibrational information. It is not linear. It is a merging with wholeness. And within that wholeness, your client's higher consciousness exists as well.

The avenue by which psychics pick up information (and where you as a healer may do the same) is through the senses: feeling, intuition, color, symbols and sometimes dreams. Very often, I will receive information for a specific client I'm working with in a dream.

Channeling information is natural meditation by the 3rd eye. It has been recognized for thousands of years as an opening or unveiling of the barrier between our conscious and super-conscious.

If you're reading this, then you are already aware of the universal mind, either consciously or subconsciously. The general public tends to ignore the information they are given or have access to and effectively sleepwalk through their day by simply *re*acting, rather than taking an active role in their lives. This knowledge is an alarm. You may try and hit snooze, but it will keep on buzzing until you wake up. So turn off the alarm. Keep a journal by your bed to write down any dreams. Keep a notebook or pen and paper with you during the day and start jotting down those random thoughts. The connection is always on. The channel is always open to some degree. When you become distracted or detached, you can always find it again. Simply quiet your mind and it is there.

How to Channel

Before *every* healing technique, use this imagery to lift your vibrational states so you can help lift your client's vibration. If you're in a bad mood, tired, or busy-minded, then balance yourself first with the Chakra Imagery. You must be focused and centered to ensure you are offering your client a clear, clean and true healing.

- Sit at the clients head with your palms approximately 1 foot above their crown chakra, imagining a ball of white light.

- Channel the divine spirit (Gods love and light) into this ball of chi. You are establishing a connection to *their* higher source.

- State your intention (i.e. "I ask to be the perfect channel from the highest vibration of love and light to____(name of client)____for his/her highest good in body, mind and spirit. You may create your own intention of prayer to make it more personal to you.

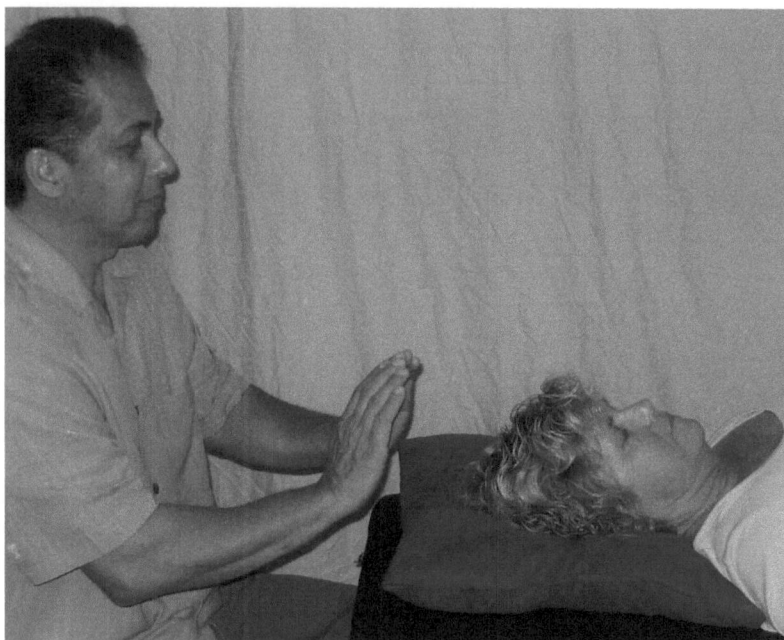

Channeling Correctly

Sometimes its difficult to keep your channel open for the duration of a healing treatment. The usual reason for this is that *you're trying too hard*. It takes a long time, even years, to establish and understand your relationship with the source.

Much like any relationship with yourself or another, the relationship between the higher source and you will grow and evolve over a lifetime. And, as in any relationship, you will understand each other more in time and learn how to connect more easily. The first step is getting acquainted. Who am I in relation to you? Who are you in relation to me? Who are we as a team?

At some point, you will go through your own power/ego struggle. Therein lies a trap. The ego will want to take over and use your own energy for the healing rather than channeling it from the divine source. Remember, *you* are not healing them, *God* is. When you try to use your own personal energy instead of channeling the energy from the source, you only drain yourself of energy. Struggling with the ego is a natural process.

By making the conscious choice to channel the energy in from the source repeatedly, you will establish a clean and clear link.

You will know when you've tapped into the inseparable link to the source. It is the undeniable sense of feeling whole. Some call it "feeling the Grace of God". What you are channeling is beyond you, yet merging with you, like milk and water. The source is the milk; you are the water.

Keep it simple

- Never hold your breath.

- Let go and *let God.*

- Imagine you are the pipeline. Breathe in and open the pipe. Breathe out and open it *even more.*

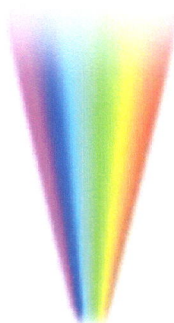

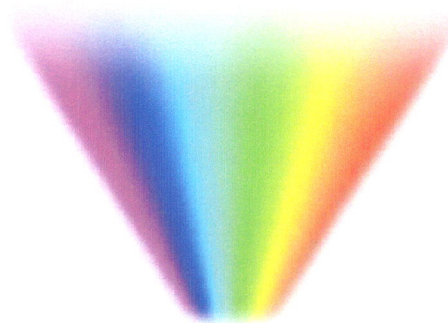

Breathe in and open the pipe   Breathe out and open it even more

Before, During & After
Every Healing

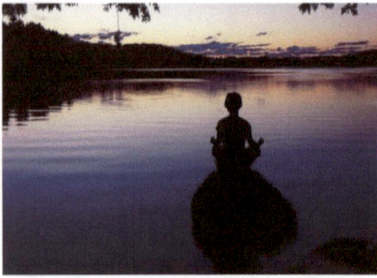

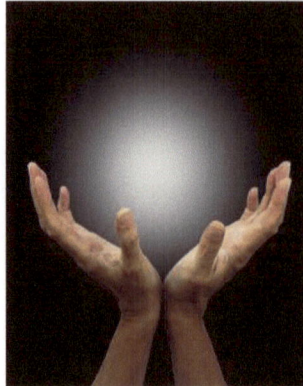

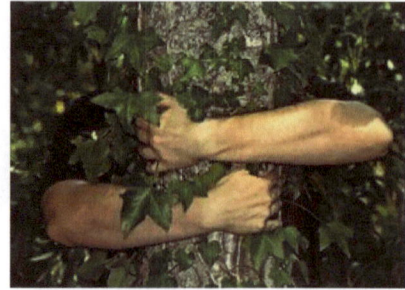

Let's begin. Here are the steps required in any healing technique.

1) Set up your altar then smudge yourself and your tools.

2) Balance and align yourself using the Chakra Imagery for the Healer (page 80).

3) Light your altar candle and say, "God/Great Spirit (client's choice), please be with us for the healing at this time. Help me be the perfect channel of healing for_____."
      (Client's name)

4) Ask them where they are mentally, emotionally and physically on a scale from 1-10, (10 being the most hurried, worried and stressed and 1 being the most at peace). This is called a "Check in".

5) Smudge your client on the table. Have them breathe in Relax or Sacred Oil.

6) Scan their aura for blockages.

7) Send white light with both palms to the 8th chakra (about 1 foot above the crown), while you establish your channel. Remember to have the mindset of unity and peace during the entire process.

8) Proceed with the healing and guide them with an imagery or meditation.

9) When completed, apply a drop of Energy Oil on your palms. Then place your hands two feet above the client's body and use a sweeping motion from head to the toe to smooth out the client's aura. Do this three times. The reason for this is to re-establish their auric field.

10) Bubble them up by using your arms to imagine wrapping them up in a clear bubble. Start from their head and wrap to their toes. Then wrap back up the body again from their toes to the head. The bubble should be four feet above the body. This is to re-establish the person's boundaries, protecting them from any outside negative influences and holding the healing in. Always allow at least three days for a healing to assimilate.
      Once per week is generally a safe practice. In this case, *less is more*. Too many healings given too close together can put the client into overload. Their body cannot assimilate the energy

quickly enough to gain the benefits from healing. It may instead have the opposite effect, causing a negative reaction to too much energy. In this case, there can be "too much of a good thing". This is an example of doing unintentional harm to a client.

11)   After they are bubbled up, put your hand gently on their shoulder. Ask them to breathe deeply and awaken refreshed at the count of 3.

12)   Do the check in again, asking the client how they feel from 1 to 10. This helps them to become aware of their own results. It also teaches them to listen to their body. If their stress level did not decrease, assure them that it will with practice. Healings are interactive. Even though the client is resting on the table, their energy and the energy you're channeling are working diligently to heal the ailments being presented. Now is also a good time to give them the Imagery for Relaxation as a hand out.

13)   After a healing, you, as a healer, must cleanse yourself and re-establish your own boundaries in order to separate the auric fields between you and your client. This separation of energies began when you bubbled up your client. It is important for you to do this to keep yourself balanced. Wash your hands in salt water or rub them in rock salt. Smudge and bubble yourself before continuing with your next task. It is far too easy to take on a client's illness or energies. Also, sage and cleanse your healing room. This housecleaning is an essential part of the healing. This last step is equally as important as every other step listed here.

In Volume 2, Julie offers a comprehensive look at a variety of altar settings including creative designs to personalize your altar as well as step by step instructions to make your own healing tools.

Test: Preparation
(For Certification)

Requirements:

Please answer each question on a *separate sheet(s) of paper*. For certification purposes include the following:

- Your name
- Date you are completing this test
- Write/type out each question, then answer it.

Channeling Energy

1) You always begin the healing at which chakra and why?

2) Describe channeling energy and how to channel correctly.

3) What is the endocrine system?

4) Which chakras correlate with which glands?

5) Some essential oils, when ingested are toxic and can damage what organ?

6) You should use no more than how many essential oils in a blend?

Before, During and After a Healing

1. Why is a "check-in" before *and* after a healing important for a client?

2. Why is it important for you to log in this information after each and every healing?

3. Why is it important to sweep and bubble after a healing?

4. Why is it important for you to smudge and ground yourself after a healing?

5. Why is it important for you to do the "Chakra Imagery" before a healing?

Chapter 6

The Healing Techniques

"These things I do, you shall do and greater."
JESUS

The Rainbow of Healing Techniques

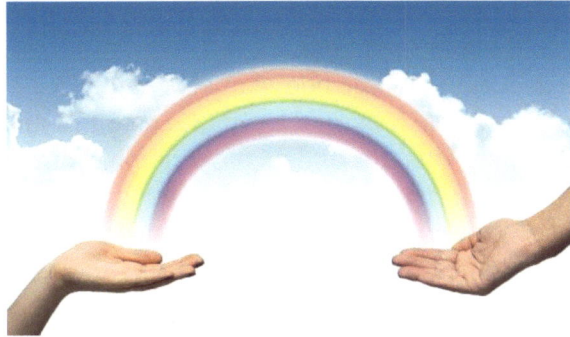

You now have an understanding of energy, aura, chakras and frequencies that are emitted in the forms of specific colors of the rainbow. There are several healing modalities, each of which resonates with a different color frequency.

- **Red and Orange:** Magnetics, crystals, specific stones, sound pitches, symbols and essential oils.

- **Yellow:** 20 chakra balancing, polarity balance, specific stones, sound pitches, symbols and oils.

- **Green and Blue:** Polarity balance, specific stones, sound pitches, symbols and oils.

- **Violet and White:** Reiki and Sacred oil.

There are also specific herbs, essential oils and chants designated to each chakra. These are all covered throughout this manual.

Each frequency/color/chakra contains a particular range of consciousness, (see "Once Upon A Time - A Chakra Story) therefore you must utilize the appropriate frequency/wave length in order to remove blockages and restore the balance of a particular chakra. This is why it is important for a healer to learn various techniques to achieve harmonic balance with each frequency as required.

The more healing tools you have in your toolbox, the more effective you will be as a healer.

The 20 Chakra Balancing Technique: Introduction

The 20 Chakra Balancing is actually a multifaceted healing technique. Aside from balancing the eight *primary* chakras (above the crown, crown, third eye, throat, heart, solar plexus, second and root), it also includes these *secondary* chakras: Shoulders, elbows, wrists, hips, knees and ankles, as well as *energy release points* in the feet and palms.

This technique not only balances the whole body but also detoxifies it. Toxins tend to coagulate in the weakest areas of the body and generally in the joints. Therefore this healing method is the most effective for: sickness, weakness, arthritis, pre and post-operation, immune system depletions and overall tune up. It also is the most effective technique when adding stone layouts, color therapy and acupressure points. Because it clears and awakens the numerous chakra locations, I have observed that energy applied through the acupressure points is received by the body system more readily.

Healings are about balancing the energies. Many people mistakenly think that a healing will increase their energy and strengthen their immune system. It does not. Healing is about balance and homeostasis of a living organism. If a person's immune system is overly active, a result can be Rheumatoid Arthritis. If their immune system is underactive, a result can be AIDS. The healing will then lower or increase the energy in the immune system as needed. A successful healing will result with a hyper-stressed client feeling relaxed or a fatigued-stressed client feeling energized.

As a healer, I try to educate my clients about this, especially those who want or expect a psychic experience from a healing. This is not something a healer should enable or reinforce. Too many people in our Western Culture still view healings and energy work as mystical phenomenon. The more you educate yourself, the better you can educate your clients.

That is why I strongly suggest that my students read our recommended book list and continue to educate themselves in the scientific basis of energy at work, especially in the field of Quantum Physics.

In recent years, much time and study has been dedicated to understanding healing energy. Through the years, scientific discoveries and explanations have been published regarding energy work, as the study of this field becomes more sophisticated.

The 20 Chakra Balancing: Tips for a successful healing

In this technique, you will always have two hands placed on two chakras on the client's body at all times. For example, one palm rests on the ankle, while the other palm rests on the knee. Your aim will be to channel energy between these two chakras until you feel or sense a circuit of energy evenly distributed between them. You may feel it as an equal pulse in both palms and a sense of evenness or balance. Once you have established this connection between these two chakras you can move onto the next chakra connection. To make the next connection smoothly, you will cross over to it. Remove your hand from the ankle, keeping the other one on the knee and cross over your palm already on the knee and use the free hand to connect to the hip. In this way you do not break the connection between you, the energy and your client, creating a consistent transition and flow of energy between the chakra points.

You will find the first side of the client's body takes longer to equalize than the second side of the body. Your palms should have remained on each chakra *no less* than two minutes and longer, if needed. The weaker the client's system, the longer it may take. Always be earnest and patient. You do not need to feel like you have to perform or rush through it.

Staying Focused

Bring yourself back to a meditative state. Whenever you feel your mind wander, remember that the prayerful state *is* the channel of merging and transferring energy. You are not transferring energy from *yourself* to the client. You are merely the conduit. TRUST, TRUST, TRUST! That is how you merge with the G-O-D energy (**G**ood-**O**rderly-**D**irection) source and the order of creation and is how the client is receiving energy from the source. The energetic vibrational merging is a very intimate connection, full of compassion and love, like a parent-to-child dynamic. It is a spiritual love being felt here. Again, you are simply the conduit.

Your vibration of harmony is what their subatomic particles are responding to in kind. If you are not in a harmonious state, they won't be either. This is your *only* responsibility. With that in mind, you take no credit for a healing. You also take no blame if the healing isn't being received by the client. If the client is not open or ready to accept a healing, they will block it. This may be done consciously or subconsciously by the client. On the next page are the step by step instructions for this technique.

>   *Note:* The diagram for the following technique shows *23* Chakra positions. For this exercise, there are only *20* chakra points, with some of them being repeated in the sequence. There are also two pressure points to be pressed before the healing sequence (one on the palms of the hands and one on the soles of the feet) to awaken the energy meridians of the body.

20 Chakra Balancing Diagram
Overall cleansing and balancing the Primary and Secondary Chakras.

To begin: Smudge yourself and your client, scan the aura and invoke a prayer of intention.

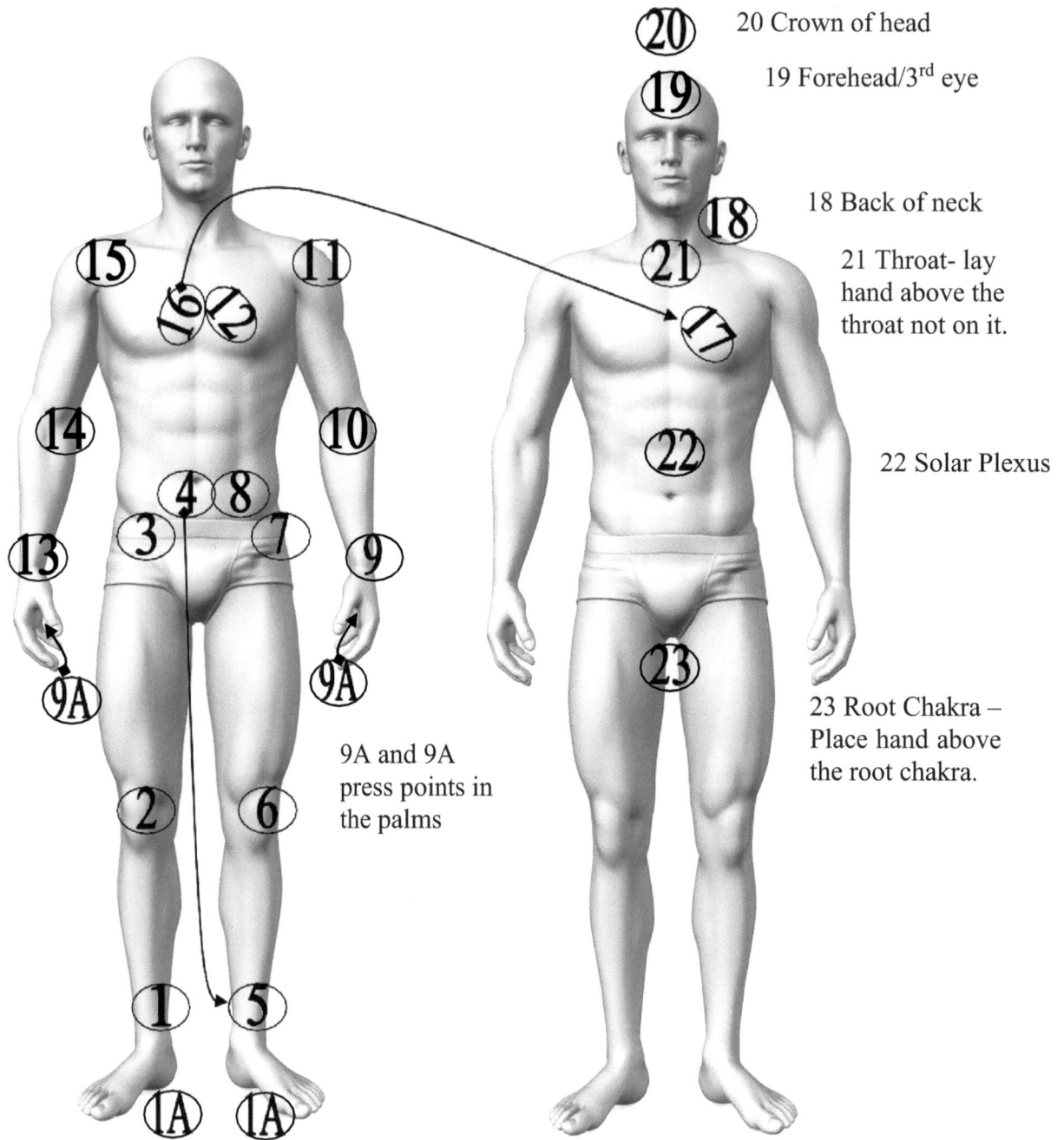

20 Crown of head

19 Forehead/3rd eye

18 Back of neck

21 Throat- lay hand above the throat not on it.

22 Solar Plexus

9A and 9A press points in the palms

23 Root Chakra – Place hand above the root chakra.

1A & 1A are at the bottom of the feet

To finish: Sweep, bubble. Give your client time to reflect and ground.

The 20 Chakra Balancing Technique: Step by Step Photos

Begin with the "Chakra Imagery for the Healer". Smudge yourself and your client, scan the aura and invoke a prayer of intention.

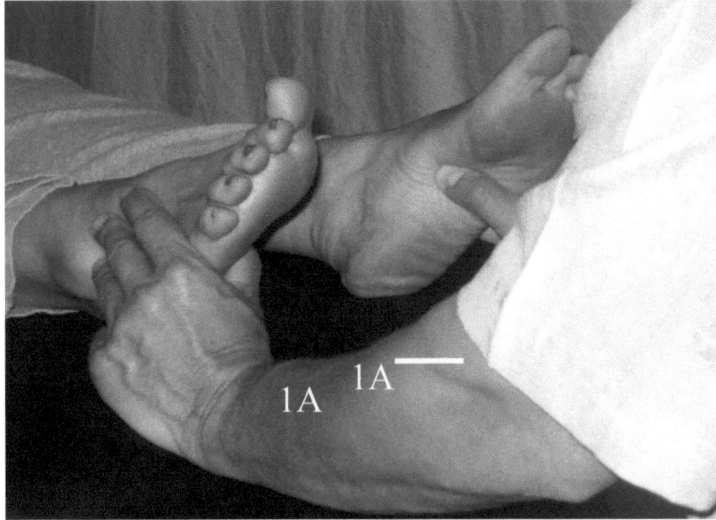

Step 1A: Left and Right side.
Press these points on the bottom of the feet to activate the
lower body energy meridians.

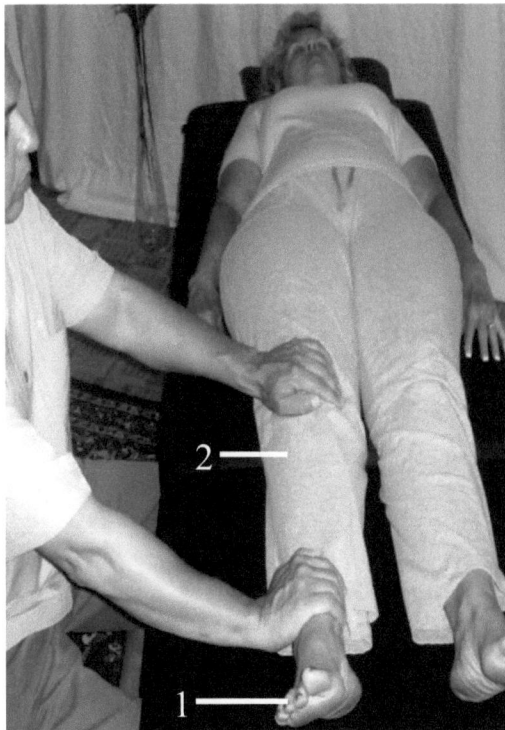

1 -2
Begin on the right side of your client. Place your right hand on
the right ankle and place your left hand on the knee to establish
the first connection for the lower half of the body.

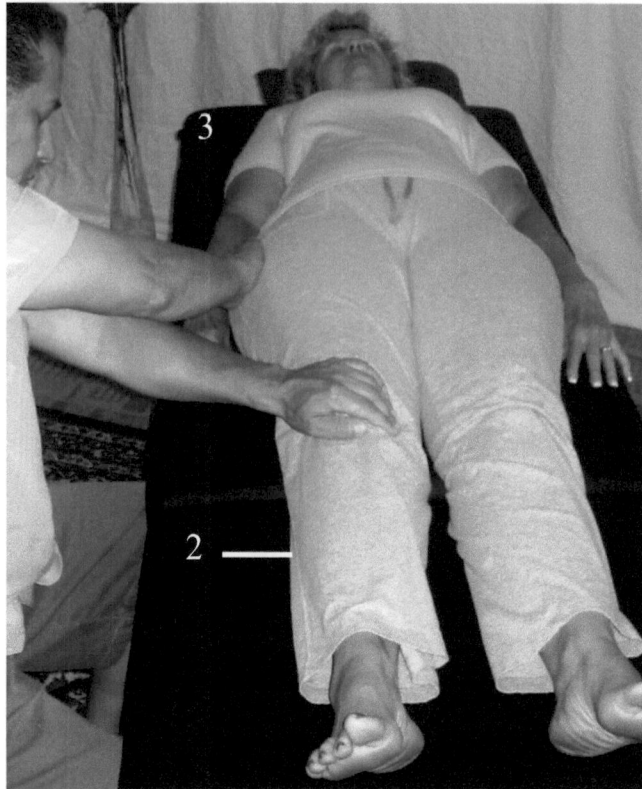

2 -3
Now gently move your right hand and cross over your left hand
and place it on the right hip.

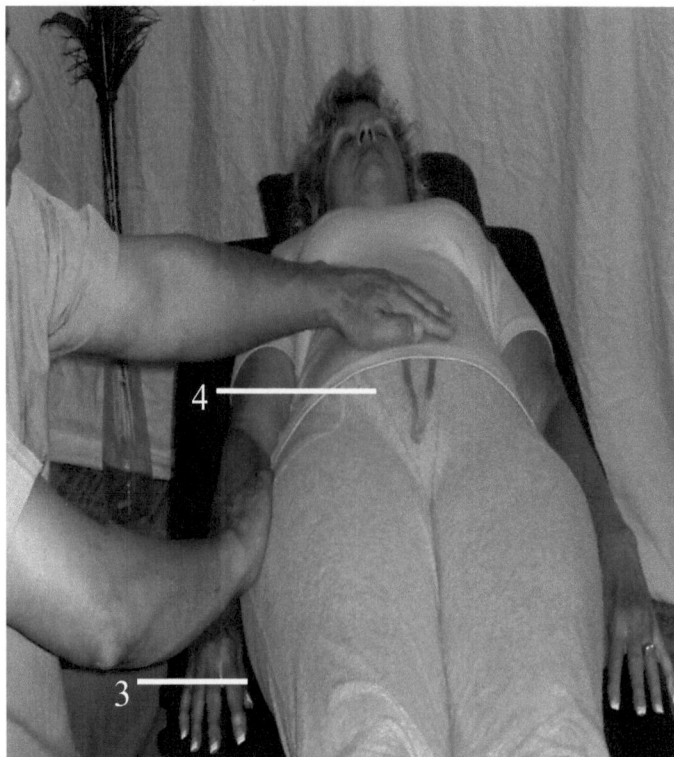

3-4
Move your left hand from the knee and lay it softly on the second chakra.
This completes the right side lower body balancing.

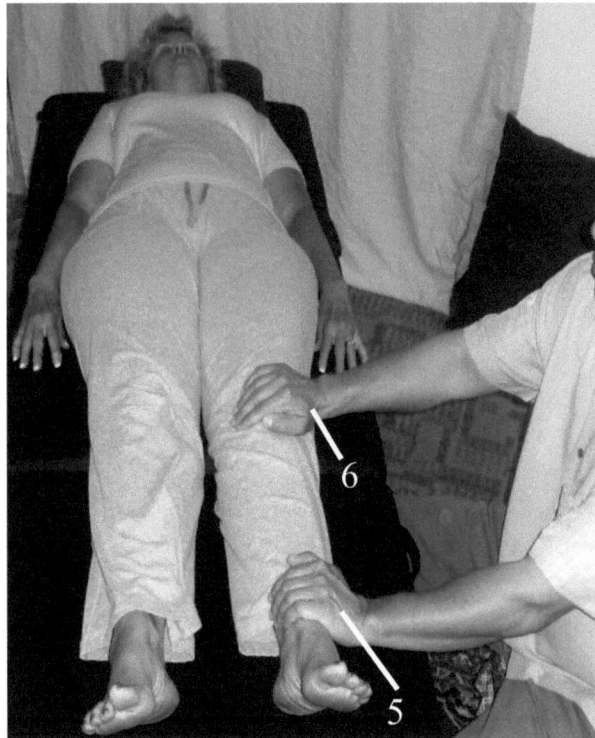

5-6
Now the left side. Place your left hand on the left ankle
and place your right hand on the knee.

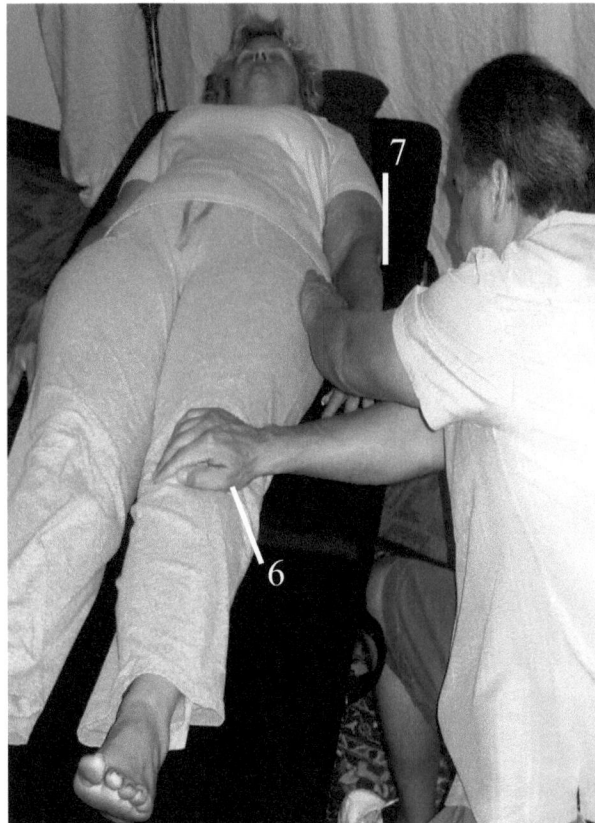

6-7
Move your left hand and cross over your right hand
and place it on the left hip.

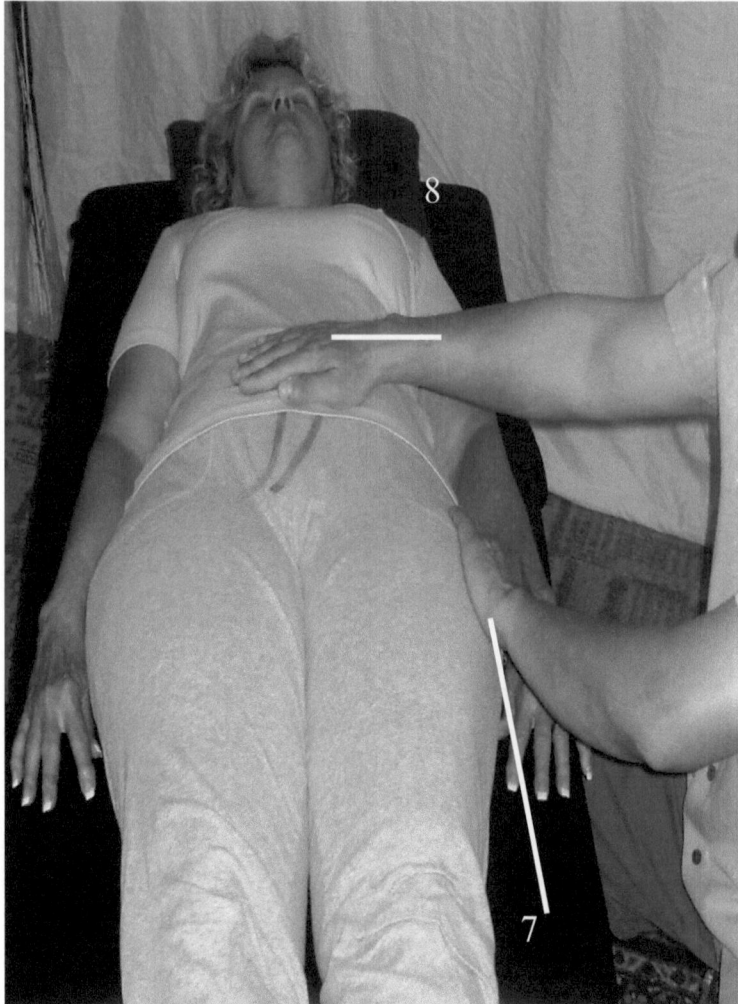

7-8
Gently move your right hand from the knee and
lay it softly on the second chakra.

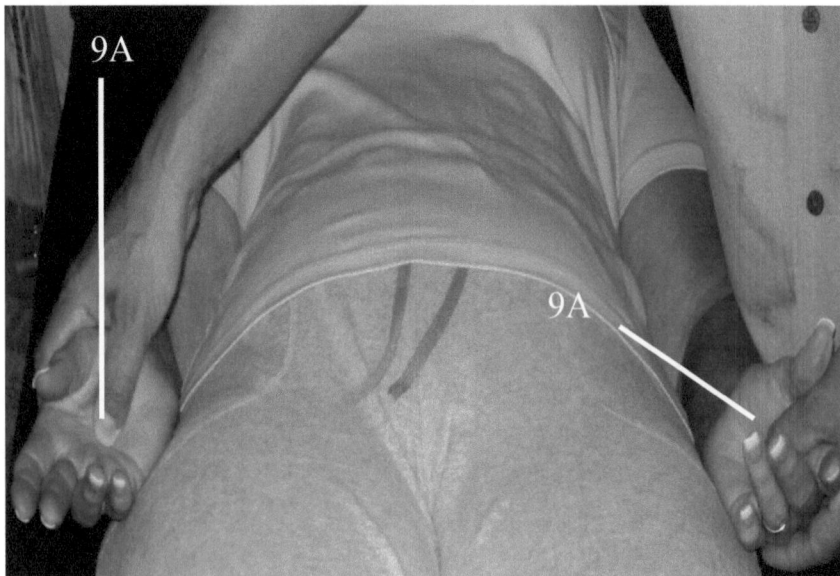

9A Left and Right Side
Pressure point in the middle of each palm
activates the upper body energy flow.

152

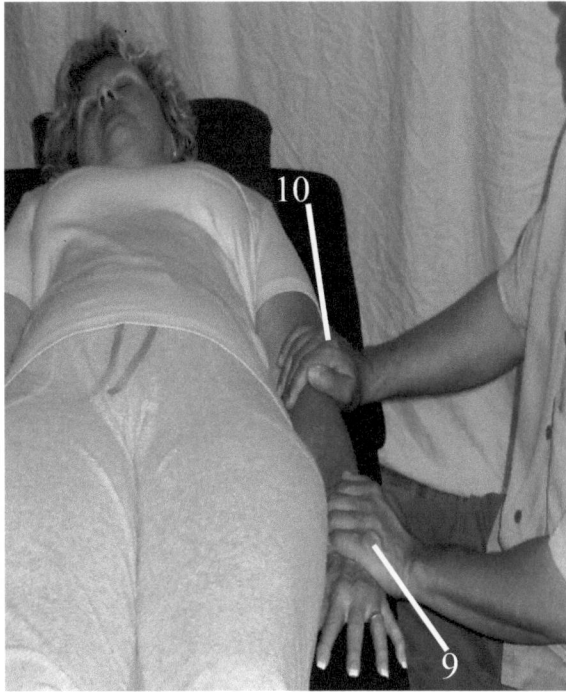

9-10
Place your left hand on the left wrist and your right hand on the left elbow.
This is the first connection for the upper half of the body.

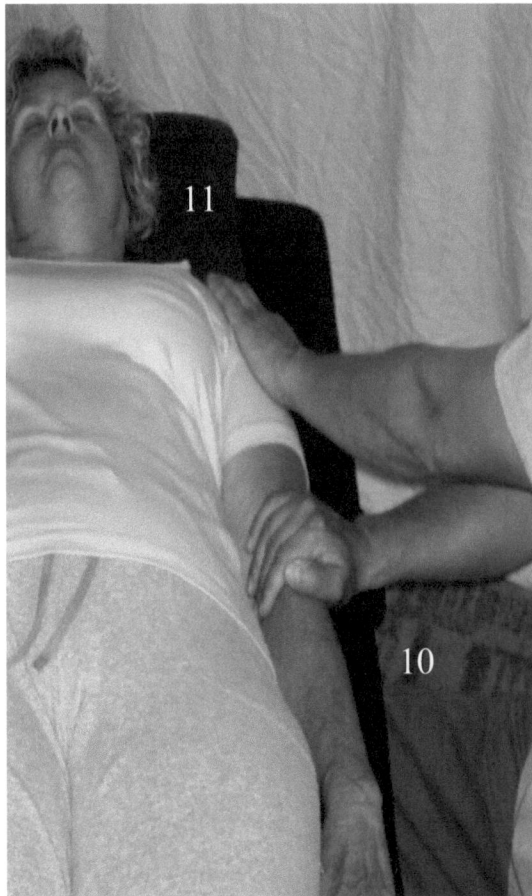

10-11
Take your left hand and cross over your
right hand to connect to the left shoulder.

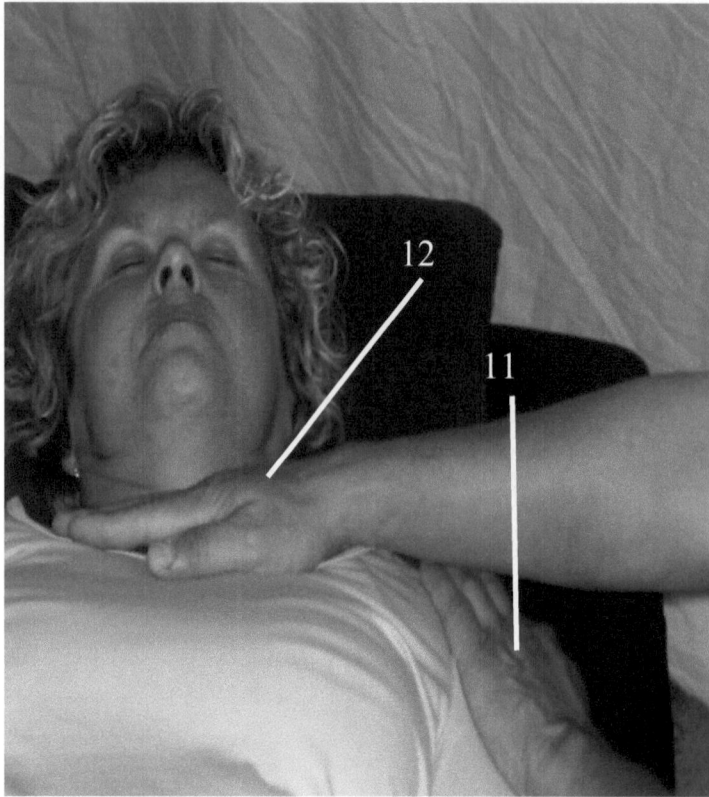

11-12
Move your right hand and set it lightly on the heart chakra.
This completes the left side upper body balancing.

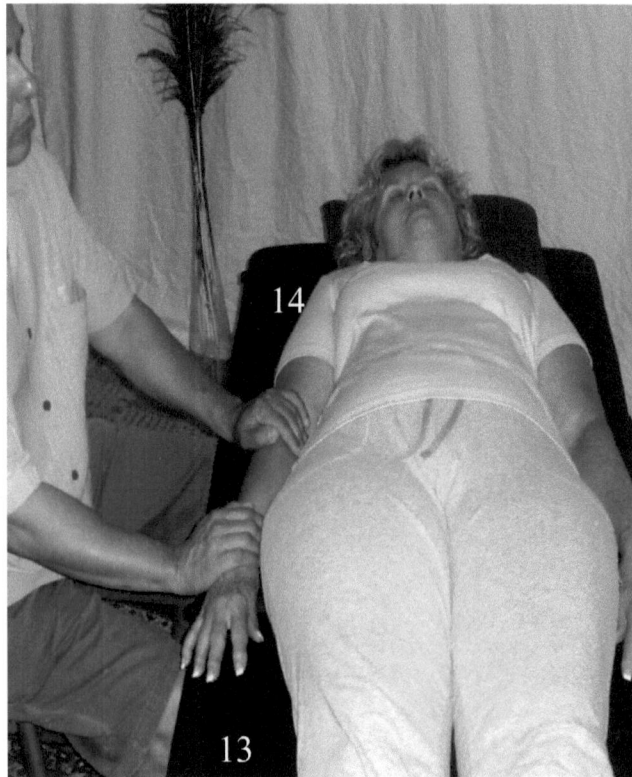

13-14
On the right side, place your right hand on
the right wrist and your left hand on the elbow.

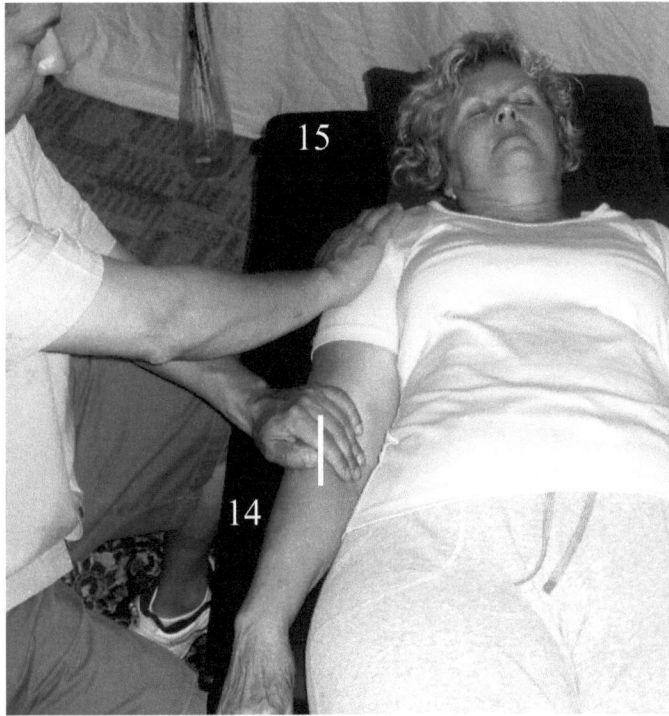

14-15
**Move your right hand and cross over your left hand
to connect to the right shoulder.**

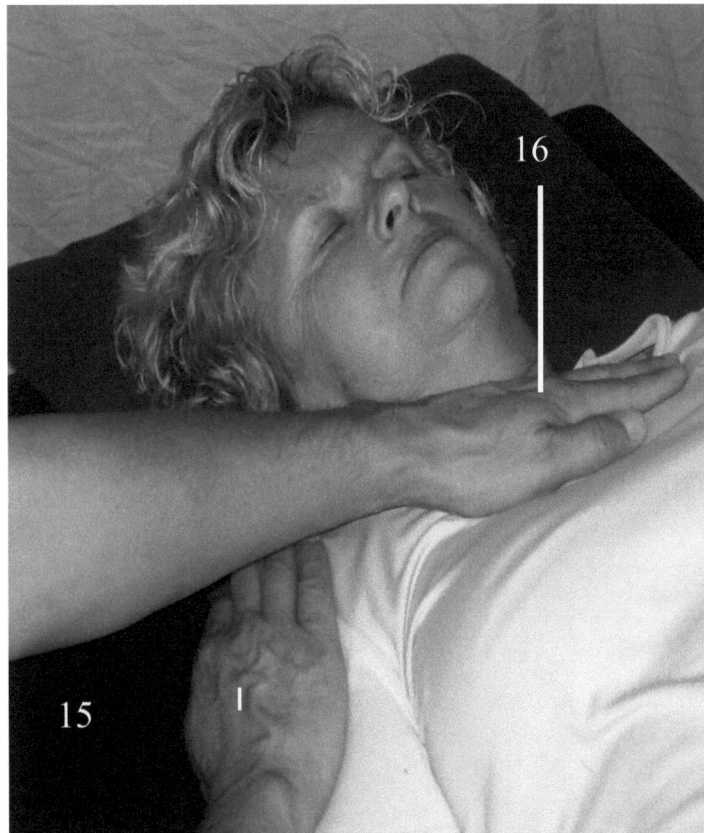

15-16
**Place your left hand and set it lightly on the heart chakra.
This completes the right side, upper body balancing.**

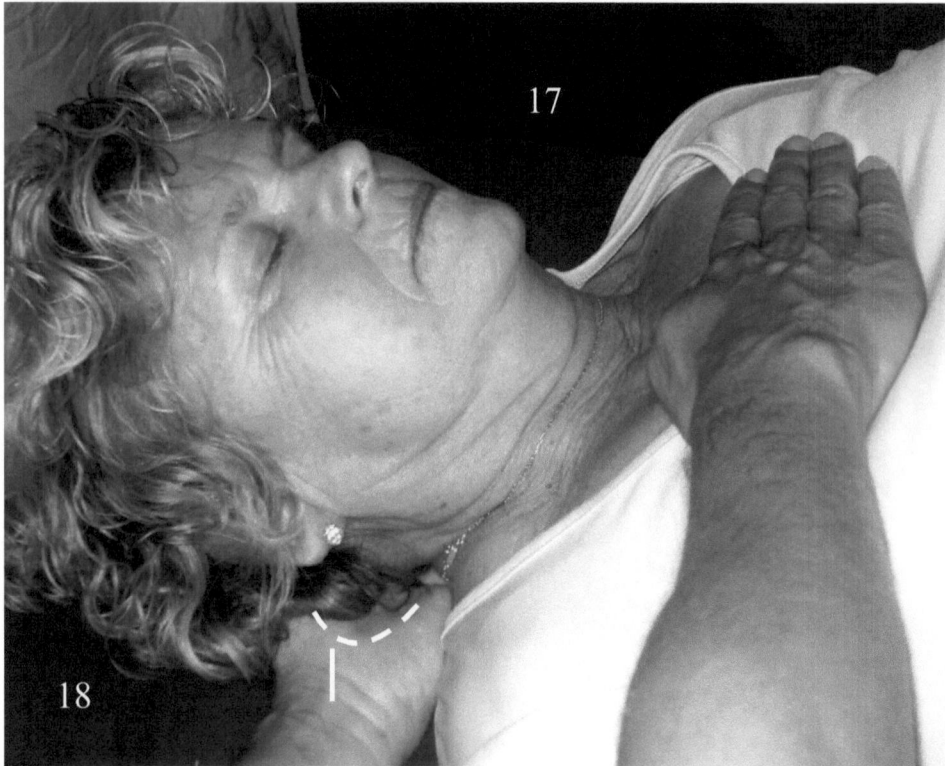

17-18
Place your right hand softly on the heart chakra and your left hand under the neck.
This is the first connection between the head and heart energy centers.

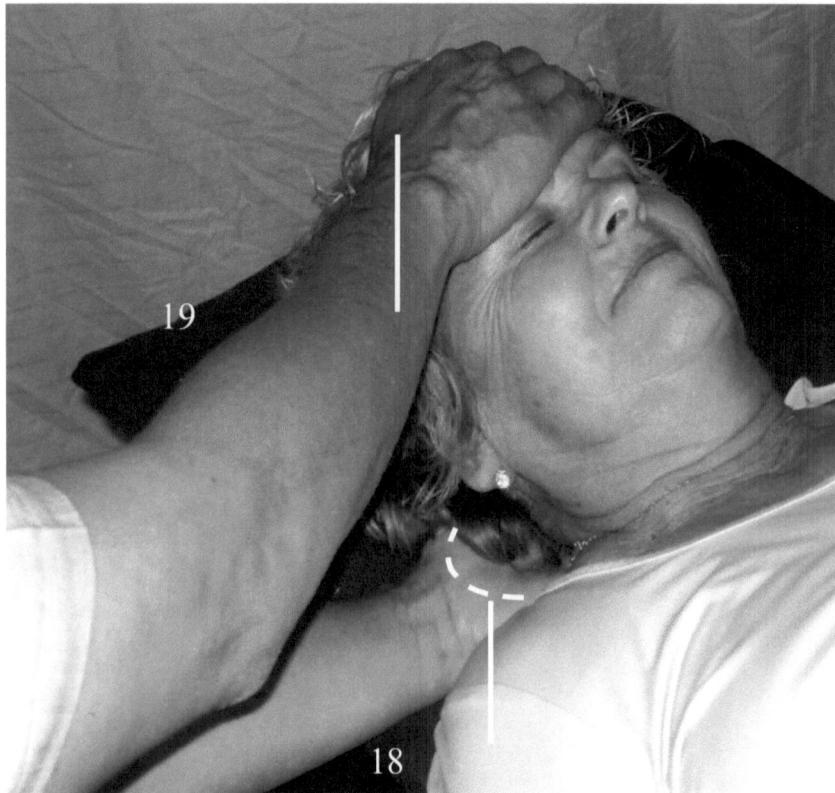

18-19
Leave your left hand under the neck and move your right hand
to the 3rd eye chakra, on the forehead.

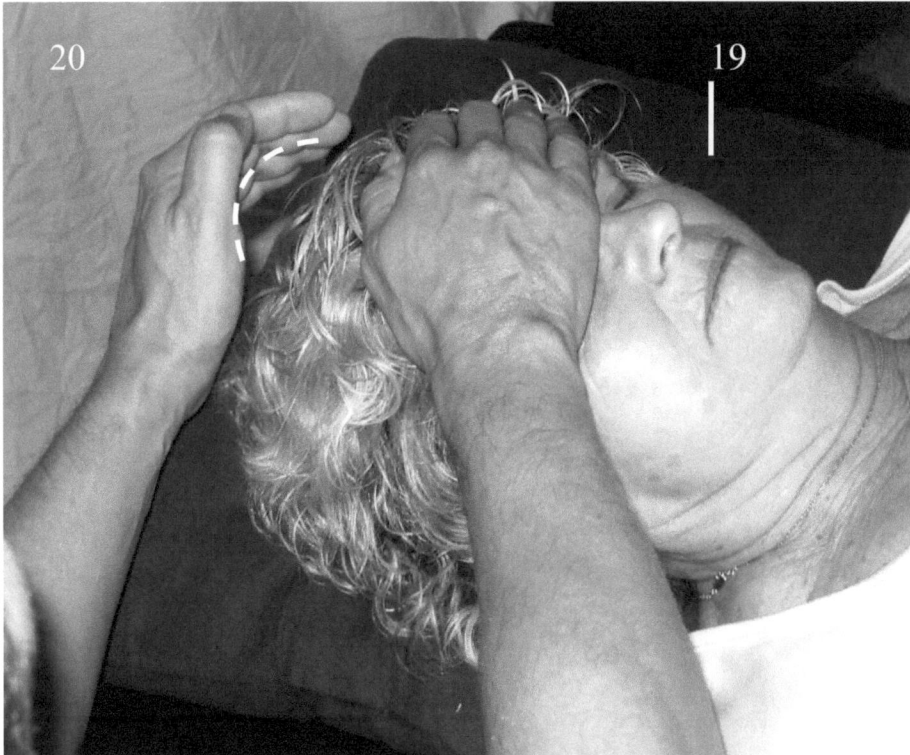

19-20
Leave your right hand on the 3rd eye chakra and place your left hand a few inches above
the client's head in the area of the crown chakra.

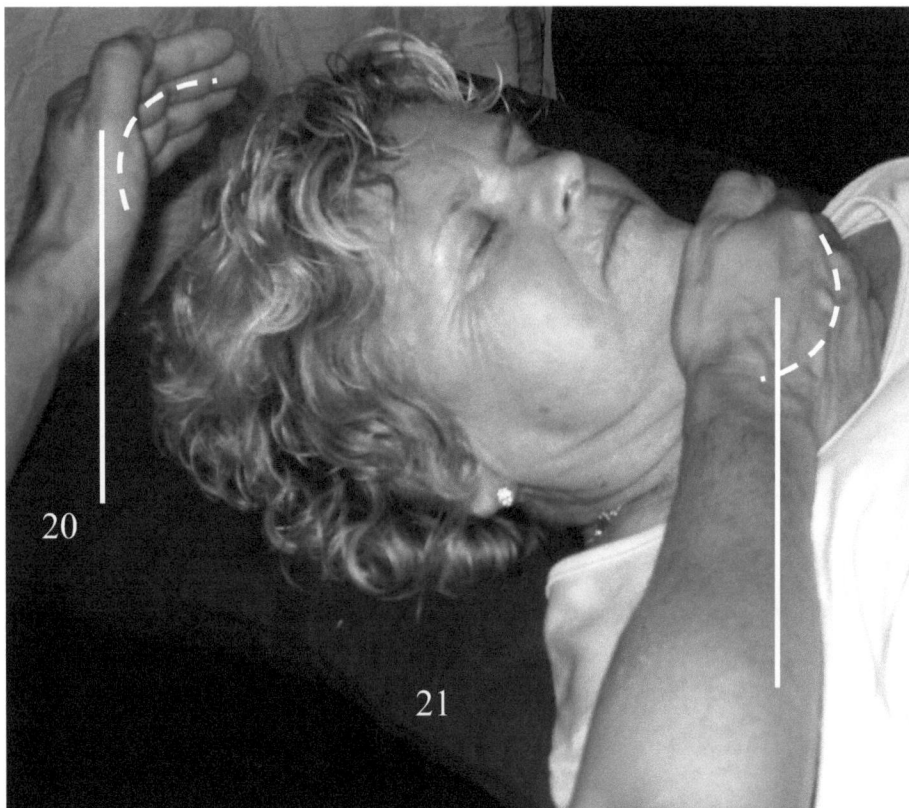

20-21
Keep your left hand at the crown chakra and move your right hand over the throat chakra.
Be aware that most people prefer not to have their throat touched directly.

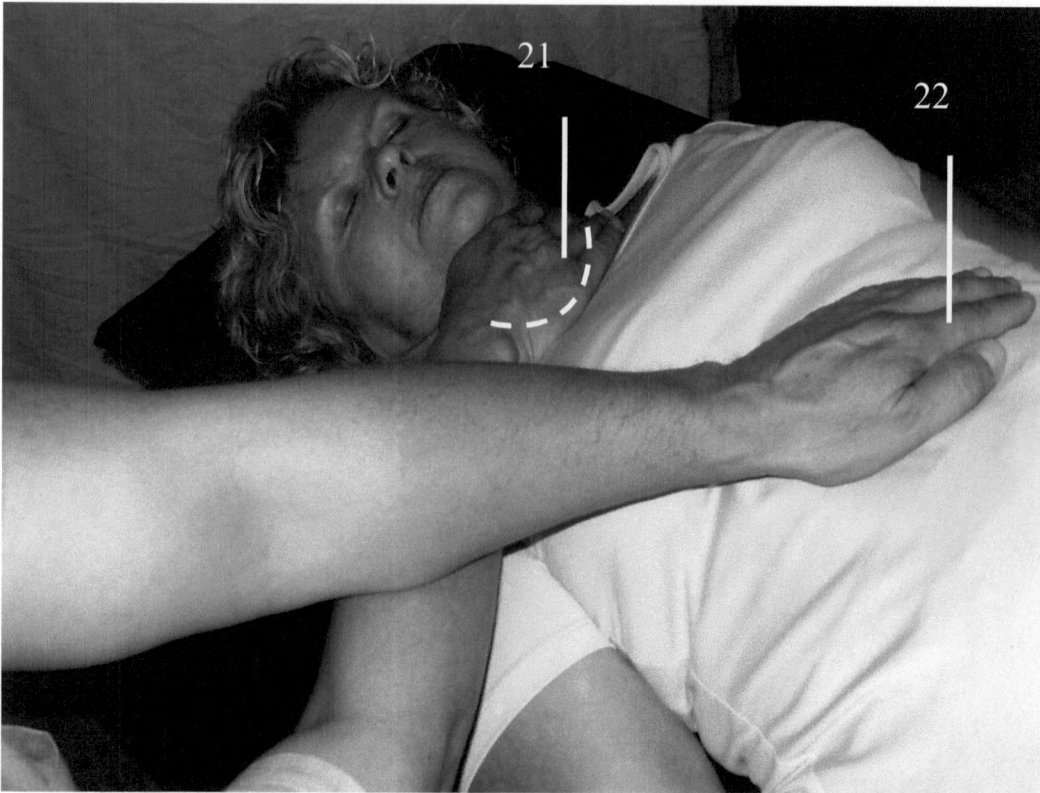

21-22
Now cross your left hand over your right hand and place it on the solar plexus chakra.

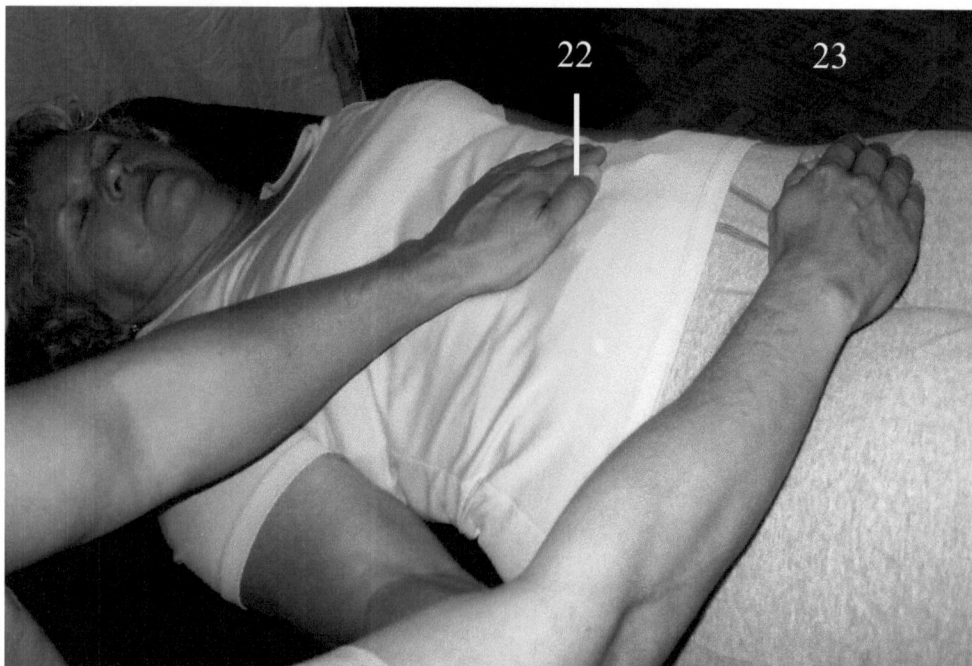

22-23
Leave your left hand on the solar plexus chakra and move your
right hand *above* the root chakra.
Lastly, place your left hand on their crown; right hand still at root.

To finish, sweep and bubble. Give your client time to reflect and ground. You may take this time
to ground yourself as well and center before discussing the session with your client.

Polarity Balancing: Introduction

A car battery has a negative and a positive terminal, or pole. The earth, too, has a North (positive) and a South (negative) pole. The human energy system has a polarity circuitry as well.

All life, every cell, atom and minute particle of energy intrinsically moves toward a state of balance. When any living system is imbalanced, anomalies are produced. In a human being, these anomalies present themselves as illnesses.

Chinese medicine and philosophy teaches the yin-yang principles of these interactions of opposites and that this is the natural order of the universe propelled by life force (Chi). It is no coincidence that one imbalance of the brain chemistry is call *Bi-Polar*.

If you were to view the human body as a universe, it would consist of numerous galaxies, solar systems, novas, black holes and endless complex interactions of energy. This energy is in constant re-creation, movement and change. It is a living thing. Energy will eventually fulfill its need to grow, flourish, build and transform to become matter and substance. That configuration as an atom, cell, mineral, planet, plant, or human body is energy coalesced through a partnership of polarities. We are a microcosm of the universe.

There are numerous locations in the body where a healer can help to restore the balance of the body, mind and emotions and numerous techniques a healer might use. One example would be acupuncture. Acupuncture's main focus is doing just that: restoring the energy meridians (or pathways) to their proper, river-like flow by releasing blockages (or dams). There are many causes of an obstruction to the meridian: physical injury/trauma, unhealthy diet, prolonged mental negativity, toxins, grief and other factors

All stresses create *dis-harmony* and eventually *dis-ease* if not addressed. The river of energy flowing through each of us ebbs and flows, weakens and strengthens, develops blockages and is always in movement, meandering through changes. Stagnation and resistance to change will contribute to dis-ease. They are directly related to one another.

How many healings a client may need depends on their condition and the degree of healing received, as well as the client's willingness for, or resistance to, the healing. Treatments are a combined effort between you and your client. I usually suggest a new client have three to five treatments to begin with. You'll both know by then if progress is being made.

I have some clients who come weekly, some who come monthly and some who come seasonally. Alternatively, there have been clients who have had instant results after just one treatment. At a minimum, I've found that performing a healing at the beginning of each season is very effective in maintaining wellness.

One of my clients, Jane, came to me with a seven month long rash problem. The rash covered her entire body. She had gone to several doctors and tried every cream and pill prescribed with little or no results. She was referred to me as a last resort. I gave her a 20 Chakra Balancing treatment and the rash went away within three days. This is by no means usual, but it does happen sometimes. When she called to tell me of the results, she asked if this could be a result of the placebo effect. I answered, "Well, if it is, isn't it remarkable how powerful your mind can be?"

Another client, Ruth, came in for a "basic overhaul", as she put it. She was fatigued and stressed, wanting hypnotherapy and a healing session. I gave her a Polarity Balance treatment with Color Therapy. I then placed quartz crystals around her root chakra, after finding a block while for scanning for anomalies in her aura.

She called me the following day, astounded. Aside from feeling generally better, a golf-ball-sized cyst she had had for 20 years had completely dissolved. You never know what to expect. That's why it's best not to have any expectations at all. Just let God do the work.

In my 25 years as a healer, I have had many such great experiences and as many with varying success. I do not question why some people heal quickly while others don't because there is no formula. Even if someone is open-minded, that doesn't mean they will heal more quickly or thoroughly. Sometimes, dis-ease won't heal until they have learned the mental or spiritual cause behind it.

Sometimes the cause comes from unresolved trauma in a past life carried over to the present. In these cases, a hypnotherapy session can help (this topic will be discussed in more detail in a later chapter). Western medicine is still in its infancy regarding the connection between body, mind and spirit. Rarely are doctors trained in holistic measures for healing the body in conjunction with the mind and spirit of a patient.

In Eastern Medicine, the medical practice has for centuries recognized and addressed the human being as a whole. There is no separation between the mind body and spirit. They are all interconnected and interdependent on one another for overall wellness.

In summary, a healing is not limited to just the physical body.

Polarities of the Body

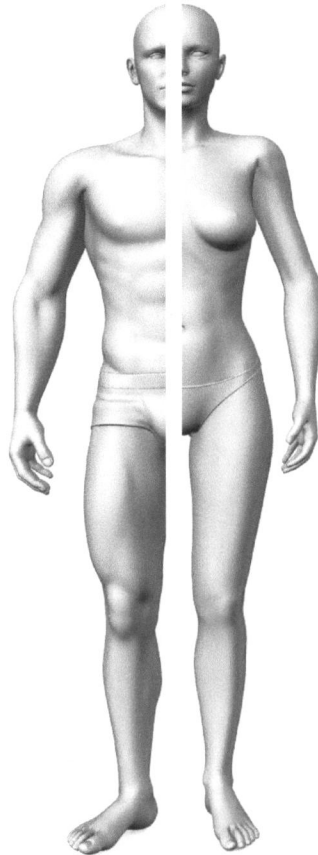

Each quadrant of the physical body: right and left, front and back, represent specific and counterpart aspects of the energy body.

Polarities of the Body	
Left	**Right**
Front	Back
Yin	Yang
Feminine	Masculine
Moon	Sun
Negative Pole	Positive Pole
Receiving	Giving
Listening	Projecting
Intuition	Logic
Inaction	Action
Right Brain	Left Brain
Counter Clockwise	Clockwise

When there is a prolonged physical problem on a particular side, I will share this information above with my clients. In this way they can assess if they are, for example, giving or acting as much as they're receiving or reflecting. They have always known the answer immediately.

Positive & Negative Polarity Points

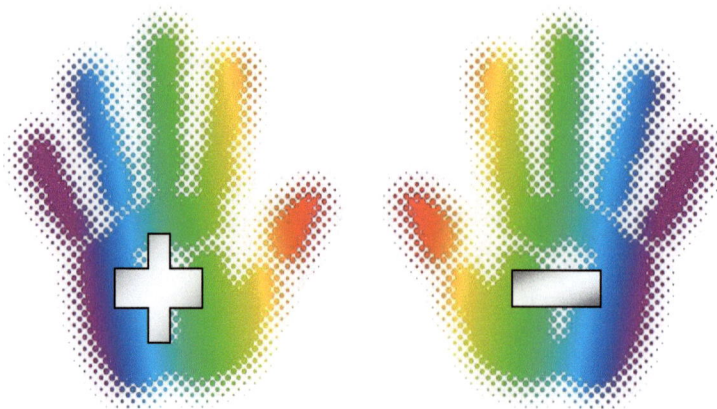

Two focalized polarity points are located in the palms of each hand. The left palm is the negative pole (receives), the right palm is the positive pole (sends). Each chakra also possesses negative and positive polarities.

In this healing technique, we use the particular polarity in each palm as a counterpart to the particular polarity of each chakra.

For example: If your client is male, his crown chakra will spin in a clockwise or positive direction. Therefore, you must sit at his right side, placing your left or negative palm on his crown to begin the healing.

In contrast, if your client is female, her crown chakra will spin in a counterclockwise or negative direction and therefore you must sit on her left side, placing your right or positive palm on her crown to begin the healing. This is considered the "top" palm.

Summary:

Male = sit on his *right* side

Place your *left* (**top**) palm placed on his crown chakra to begin the healing.

Female = sit on her *left* side

Place your *right* (**top**) palm placed on her crown chakra to begin the healing.

The Polarity Balancing Technique

Healing Preparation and Check-In

1. Light your candle and establish your mind set and intention.

2. Smudge yourself and your client.

3. Check in: ask your client where they are from one to ten (Ten being the most worried, hurried, pained or stressed; One the most serene).

4. Scan your client's aura for anomalies.

The Technique and Check-In

These are the step by step instructions. They are numbered in pairs, as this is how the healing is performed. Follow along with the diagram on the following page.

1. & 1. Place your *Top palm* gently on their crown and place your *lower palm* on the third eye. You now have both palms placed on a chakra, channeling energy. Continue until you feel or sense an equal pulsation (two to five minutes).

2. & 2. Next, move both palms down to the next set of chakras: *Top palm* on the throat and *lower palm* on the heart chakra and wait for the equalization.

3. & 3. Next, **move the palms** down to the solar plexus and sacral (2nd) chakra.

4. & 4. Lastly, place the *top palm* **above** the root chakra and the *lower hand* holding both big toes of their feet, (yes, this will be quite a stretch).

5. After this sequence, while the client rests, smudge around their aura where the chakras radiate (four inches or more from the body).

6. Place both palms simultaneously on their shoulders and wait for balance, then move on to the elbows, wrists, hips, knees and ankles, waiting for balance at each site.

7. Next, ask your client to lay on their side (*male* client on his *left* side, *female* client on her *right* side). Using your thumbs, press on both sides of the backbone/spinal cord. Start at the top of the skull, moving down the neck and the entire spinal column, pressing down into the muscles inch by inch.

8. Finally, place your top palm on the back of the neck and the lower palm at the base of their spine and wait for the equalization.

Healing Closure

1. Close them up: Sweep and bubble.
2. Ask them to check in again, how do they feel now from one to ten?
3. When your client leaves, wash your hands in water or rub them in rock salt to cleanse.

Polarity Balancing Diagram
(Overview Male & Female)
Balancing the Primary Chakras

MALE
Sit at his right side

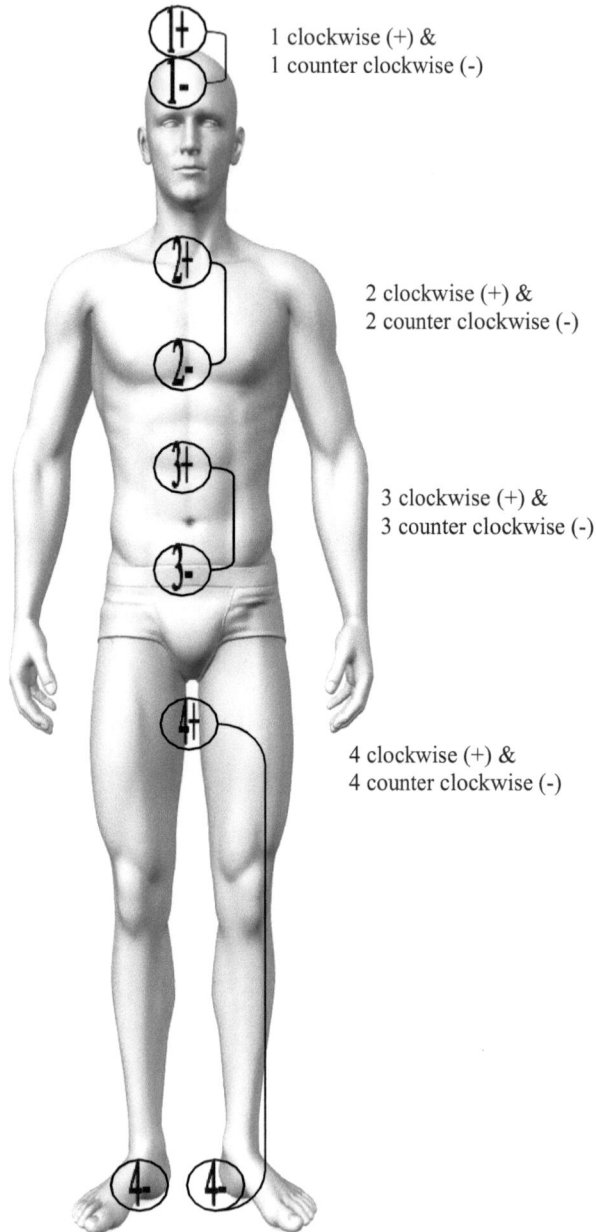

1 clockwise (+) &
1 counter clockwise (-)

2 clockwise (+) &
2 counter clockwise (-)

3 clockwise (+) &
3 counter clockwise (-)

4 clockwise (+) &
4 counter clockwise (-)

FEMALE
Sit at her left side

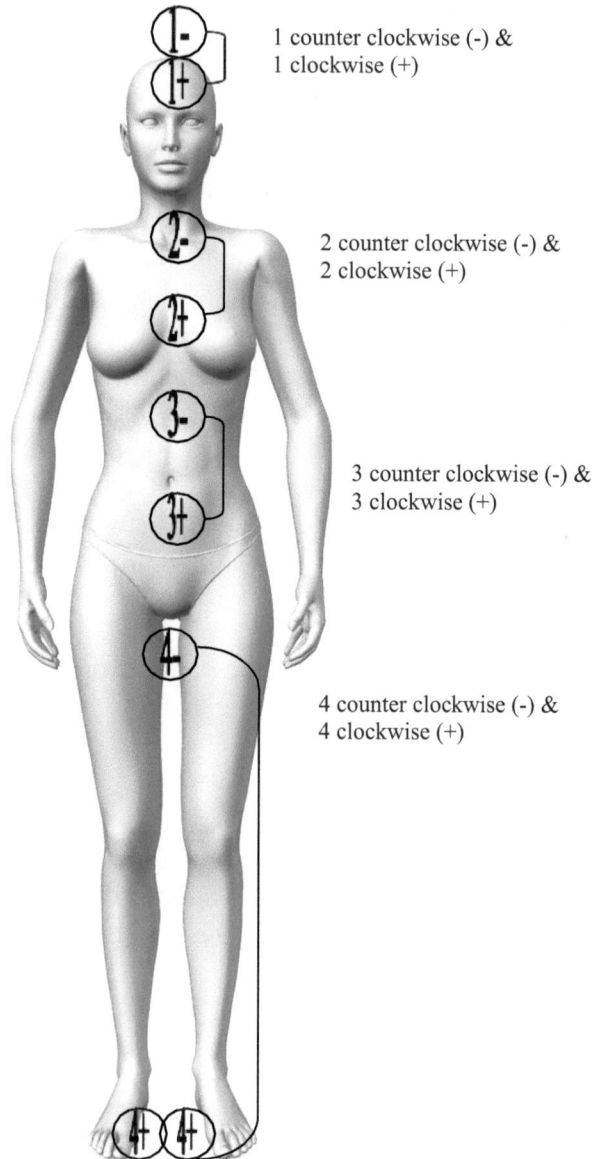

1 counter clockwise (-) &
1 clockwise (+)

2 counter clockwise (-) &
2 clockwise (+)

3 counter clockwise (-) &
3 clockwise (+)

4 counter clockwise (-) &
4 clockwise (+)

5. Smudge your client
6. End with joint balance:
- Shoulder to elbows
- Elbows to wrists
- Hips to knees
- Knees to ankles

164

Polarity Balancing Diagram (Male)
Balancing the Primary Chakras

MALE

Sit at his right side.
Begin with your
left hand (top palm)
on crown.

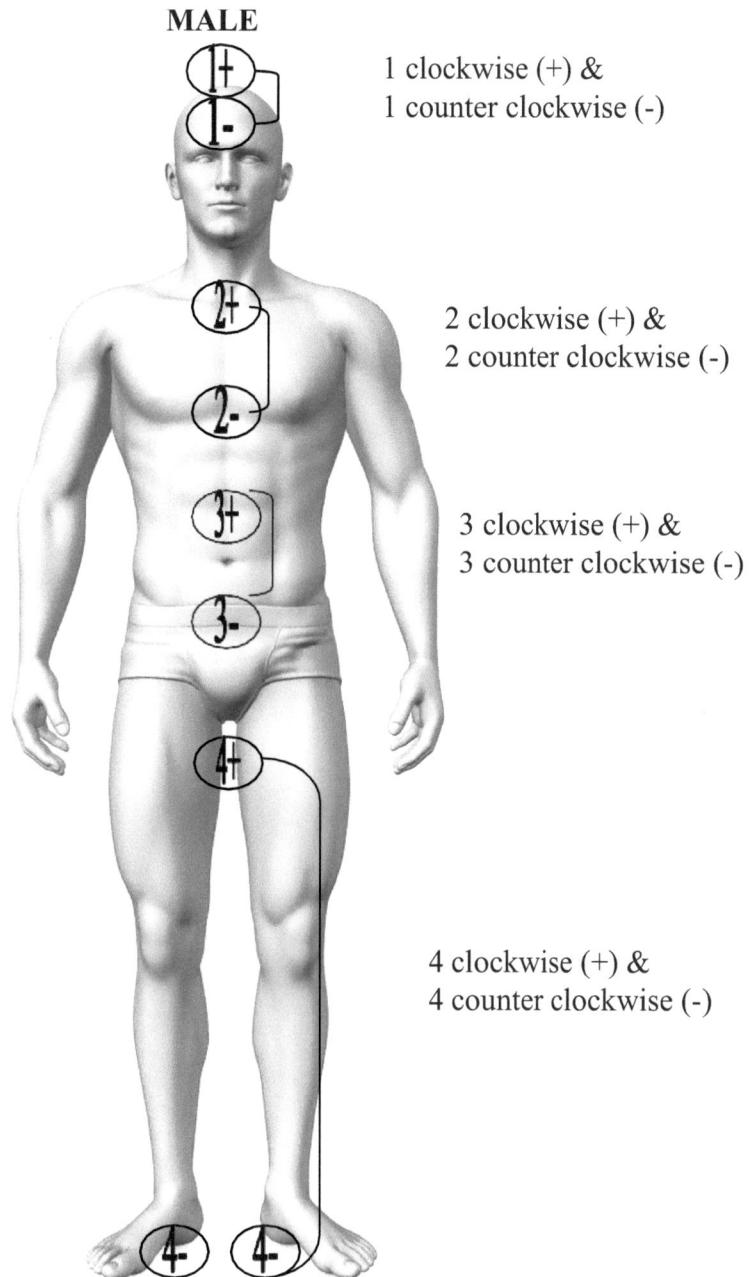

1 clockwise (+) &
1 counter clockwise (-)

2 clockwise (+) &
2 counter clockwise (-)

3 clockwise (+) &
3 counter clockwise (-)

4 clockwise (+) &
4 counter clockwise (-)

5. Smudge your client
6. End with joint balance:
- **Shoulder to elbows**
- **Elbows to wrists**
- **Hips to knees**
- **Knees to ankles**

Polarity Balancing Diagram (Female)
Balancing the Primary Chakras

FEMALE

1 counter clockwise (-) &
1 clockwise (+)

Sit at her left side.
Begin with your right hand
(top palm) on crown

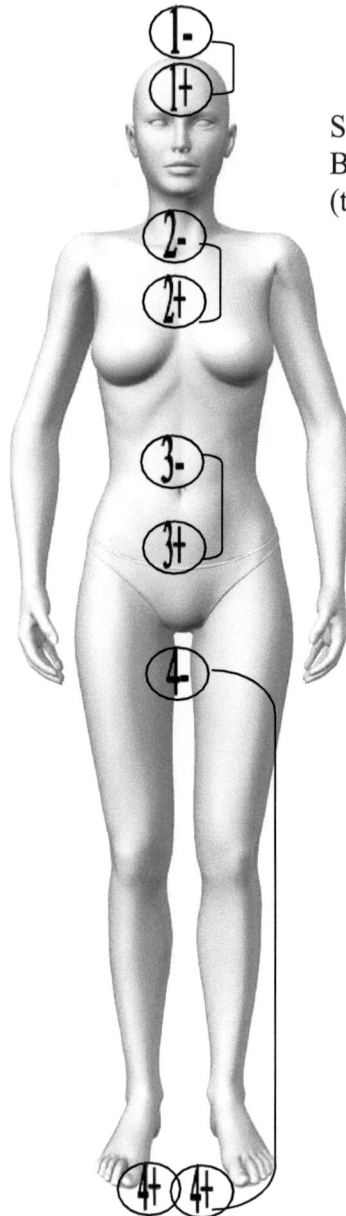

2 counter clockwise (-) &
2 clockwise (+)

3 counter clockwise (-) &
3 clockwise (+)

4 counter clockwise (-) &
4 clockwise (+)

5. Smudge your client
6. End with joint balance:
- **Shoulder to elbows**
- **Elbows to wrists**
- **Hips to knees**
- **Knees to ankles**

166

Polarity Balancing Technique: Step by Step Photos

Begin with "Chakra Imagery for the Healer". Smudge yourself and your client, scan the aura and invoke a prayer of intention.

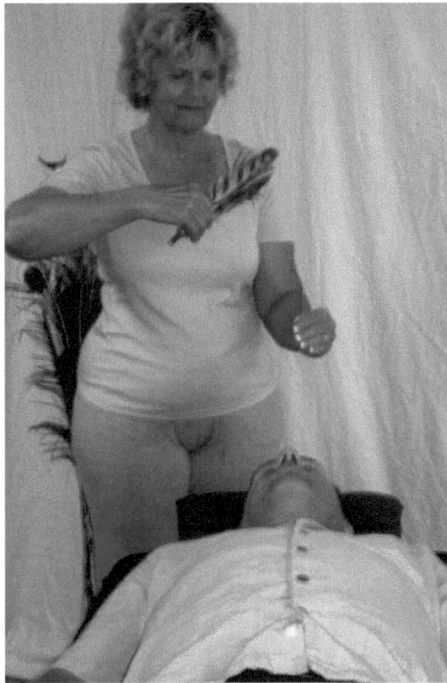

Smudging your client.

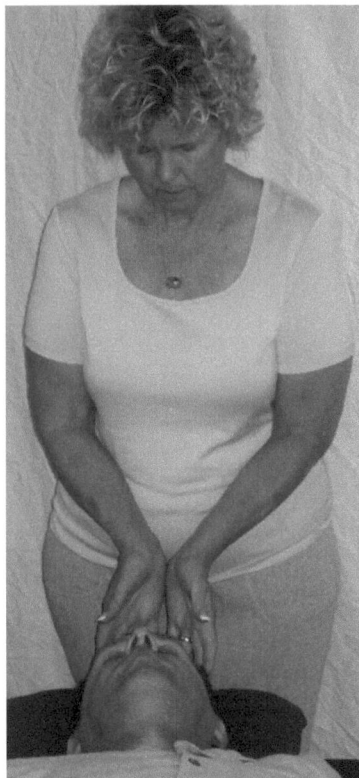

Opening a channel at the crown chakra.

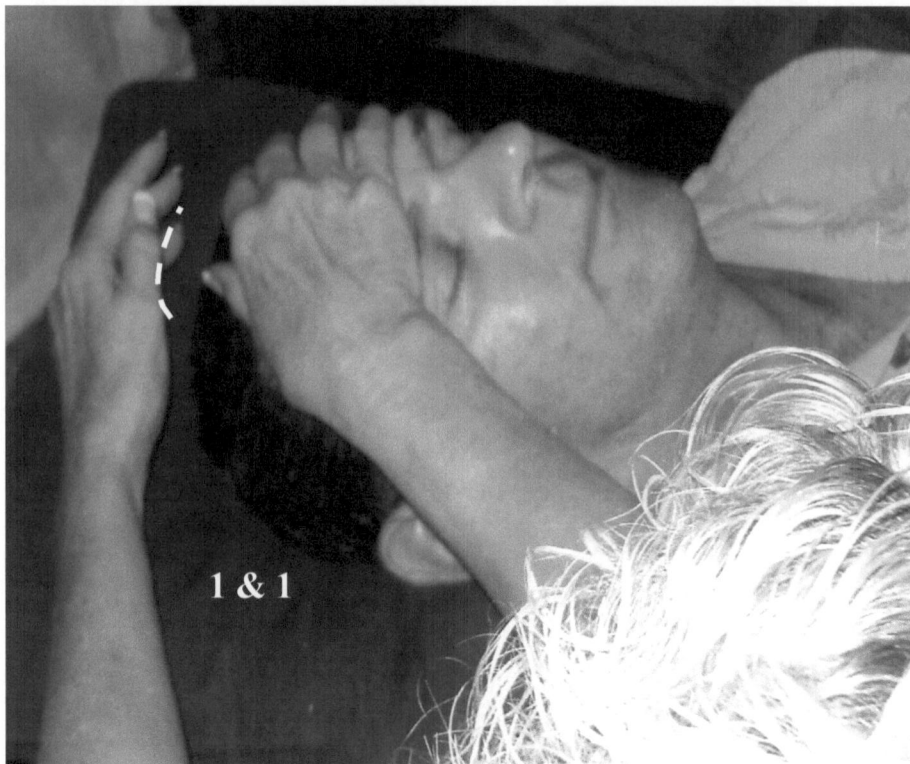

1. & 1. Place your *Top palm* gently on their crown and place your *lower palm* on the third eye.

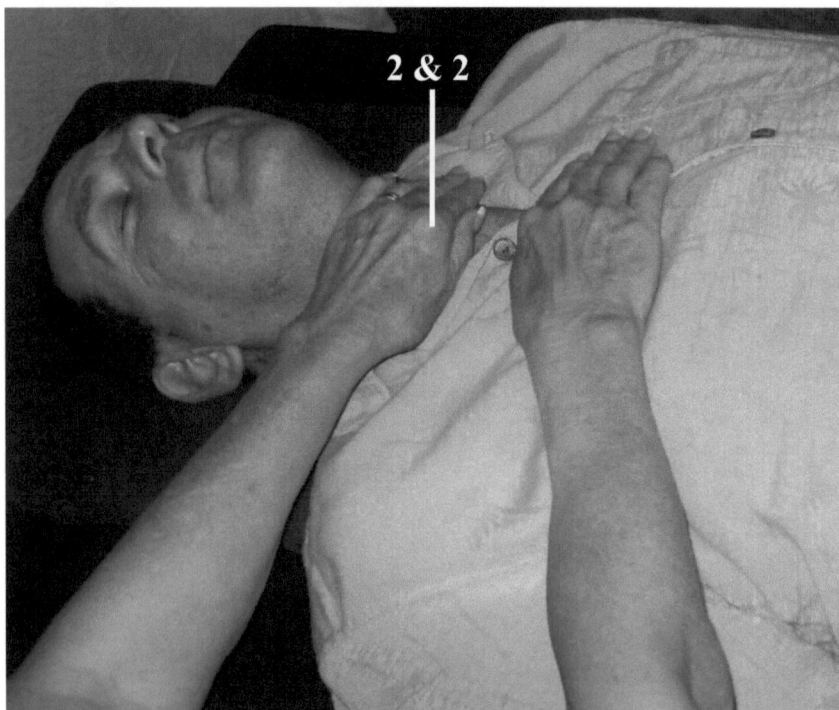

2. & 2. Next, move both palms down to the next set of chakras: *Top palm* on the throat and *lower palm* on the heart center.

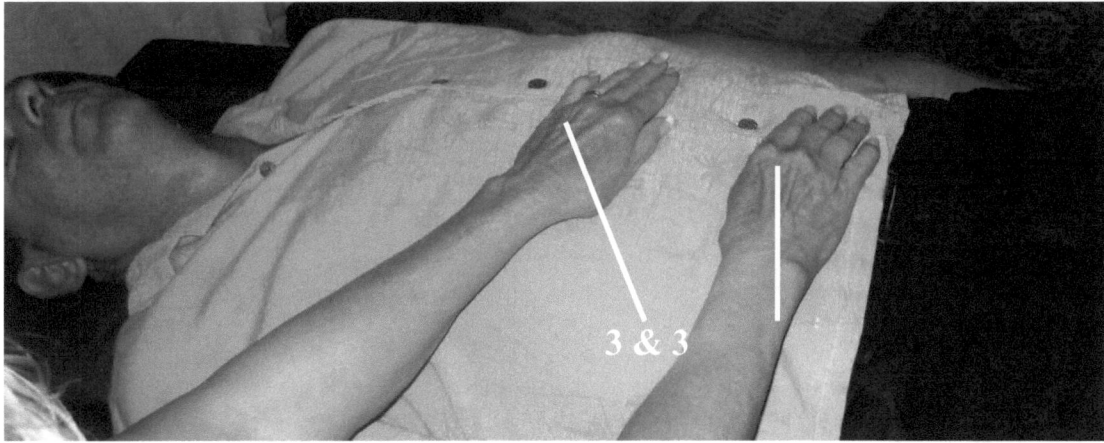

3. & 3. Move the palms down to the solar plexus and sacral (2nd) chakra.

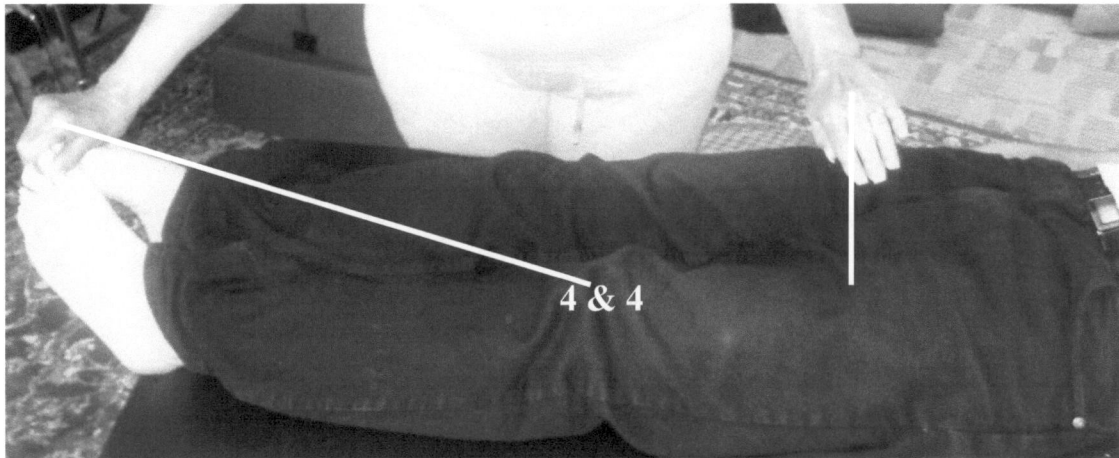

4. **& 4.** Place the ***top palm*** over the root chakra and the ***lower hand*** holding both big toes of their feet.

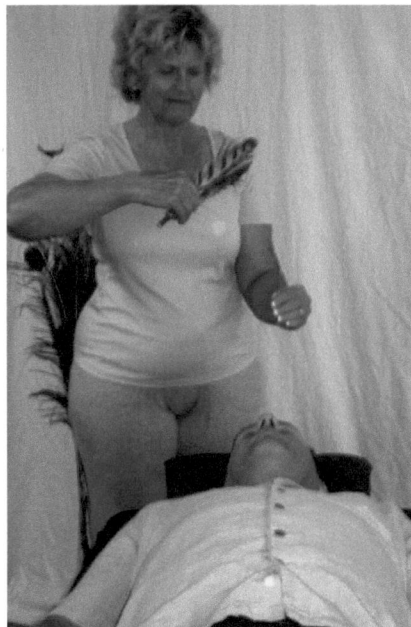

Smudge again.

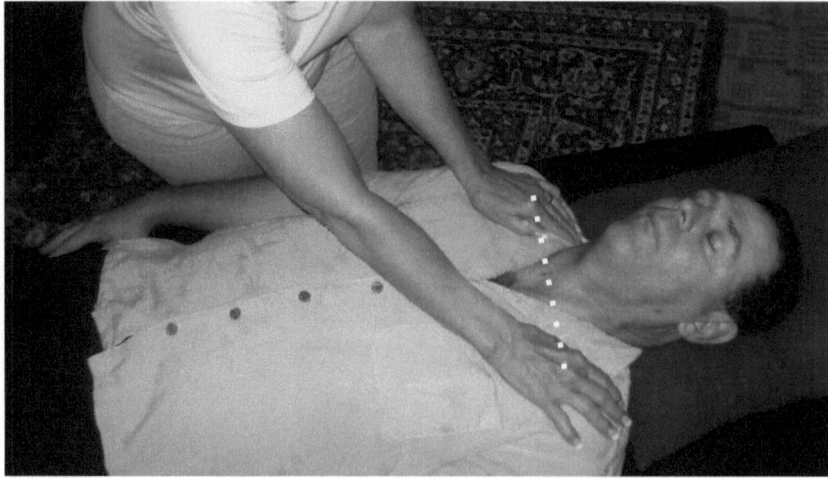

Place both palms simultaneously on their shoulders.

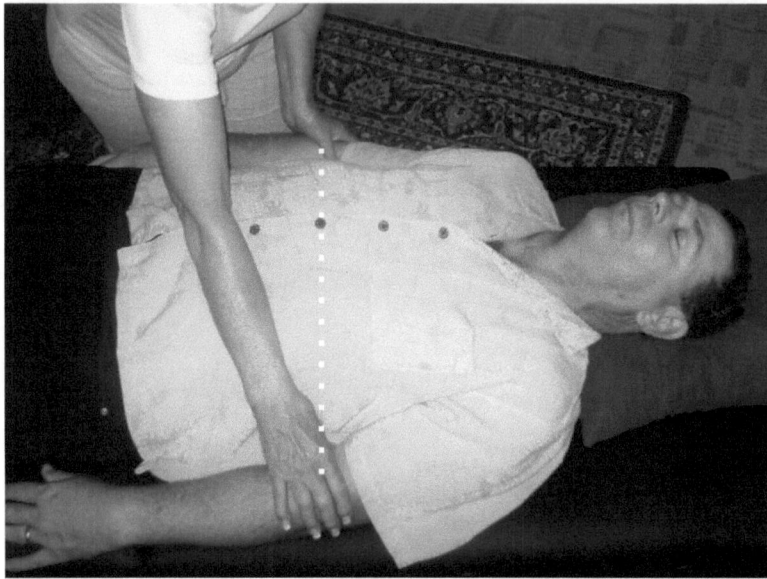

Move both palms simultaneously down to their elbows.

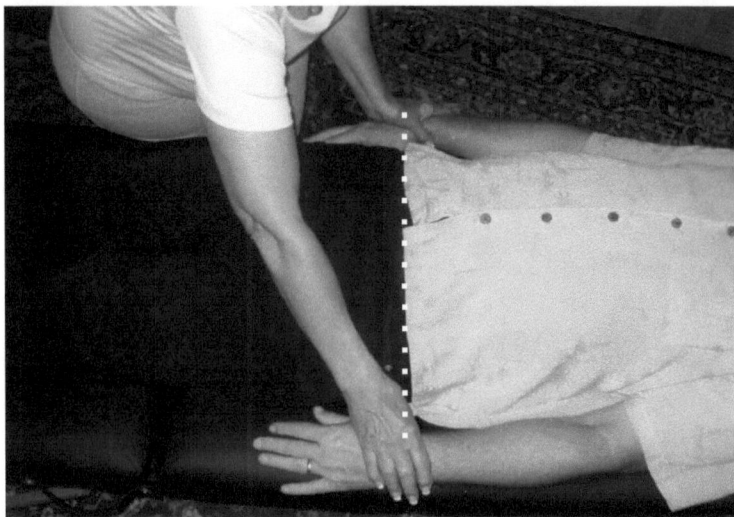

Down to their wrists.

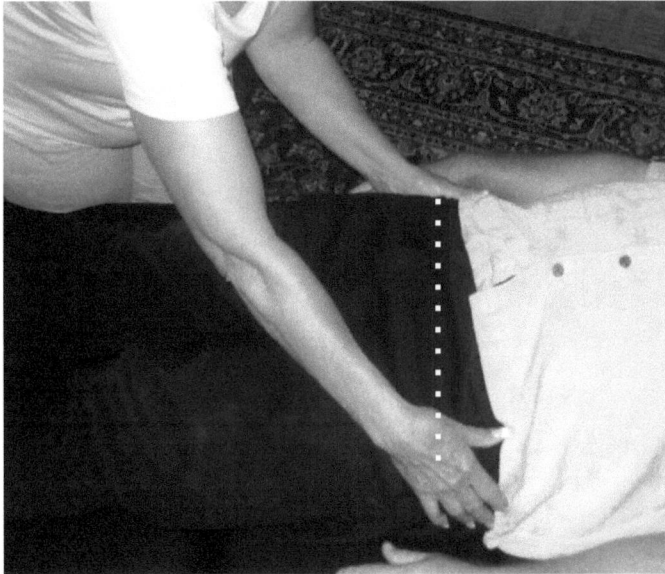

Then onto the hips.

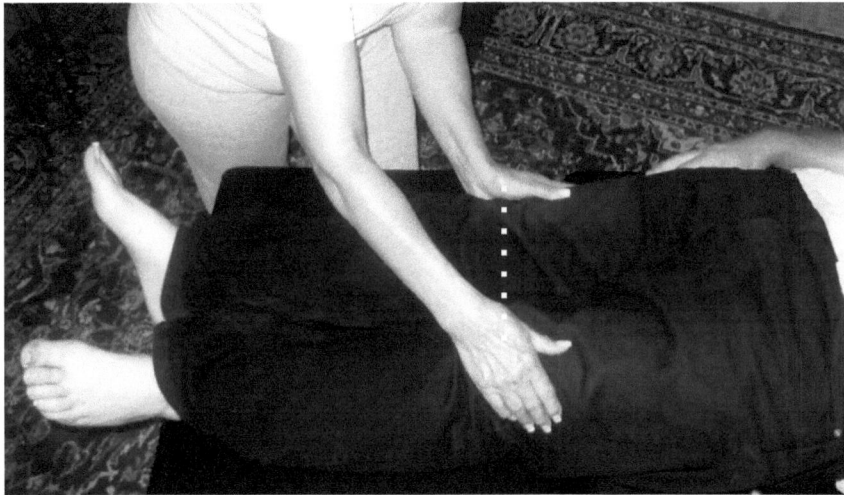

Continuing to the knees.

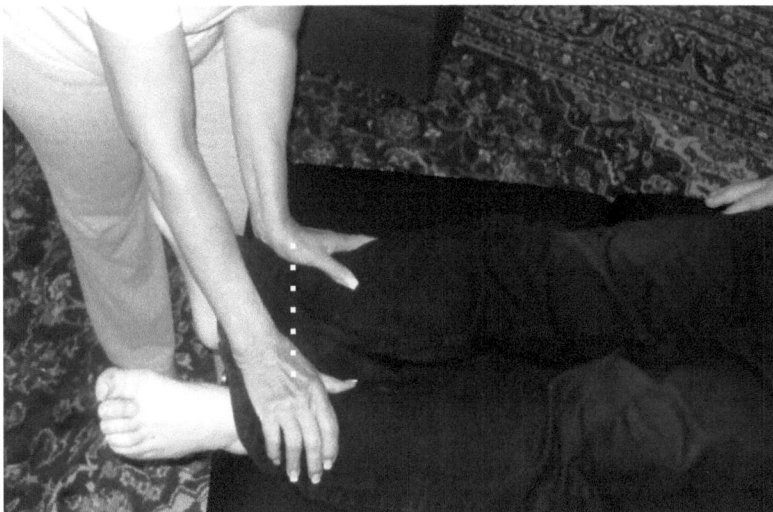

Following to the ankles.

171

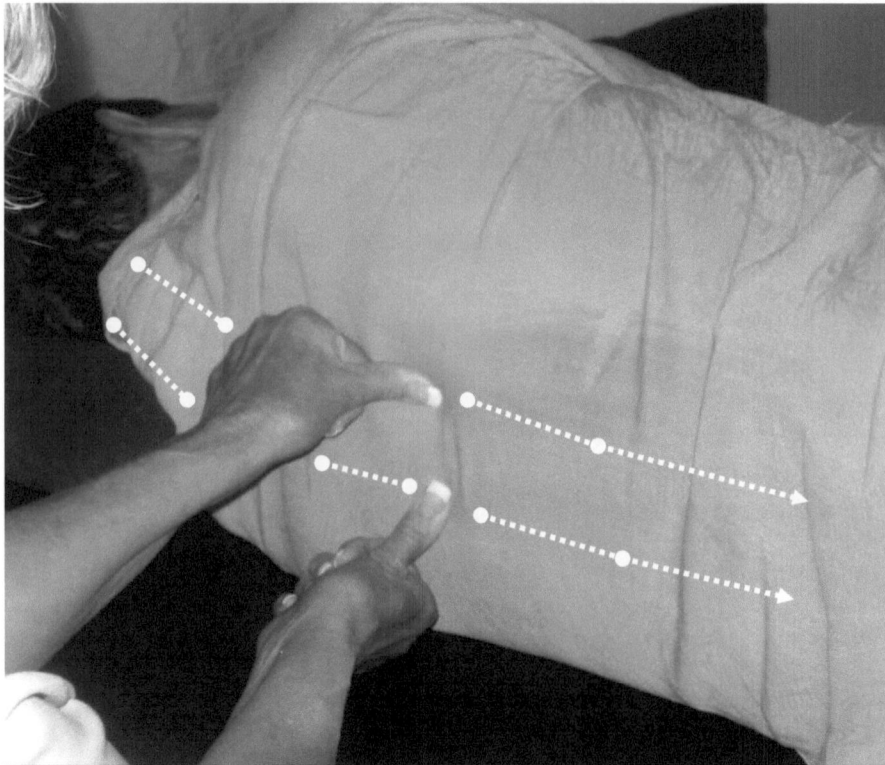

Using your thumbs, press on both sides of the backbone/spinal cord.
Start at the top of the skull, moving down the neck and on either side
all the way down the spinal column.

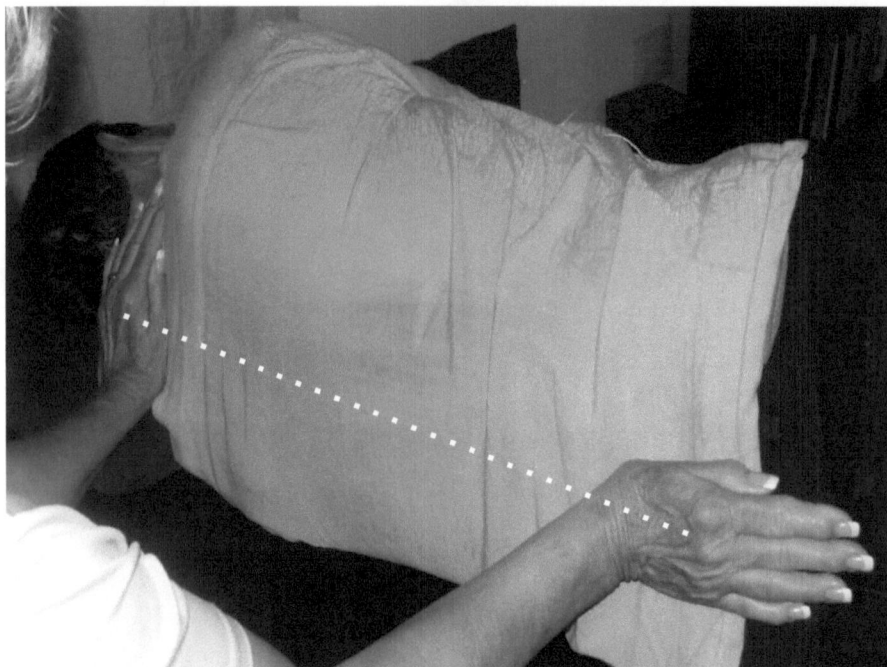

Place your top palm on the back of the neck and the lower palm at the
base of their spine. Close them up: Sweep and bubble.

Color Therapy

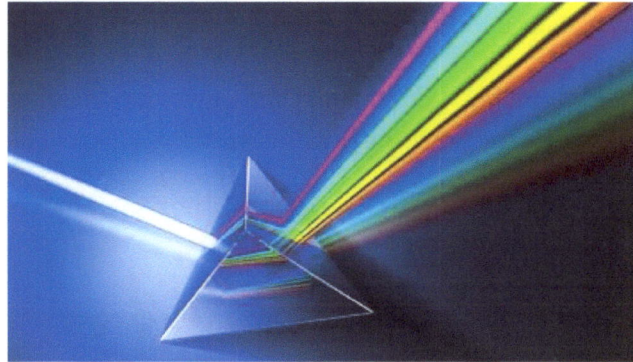

I grew up in Pennsylvania and was fortunate enough to be invited to an Amish family's home. I was 20 years old at the time, driving through Lancaster with a friend. We picked up an Amish man stranded on the side of the road due to a broken down buggy. When we arrived at his home, he invited us in to meet his family. This is how I was introduced to Color Therapy.

Inside the horse stable was a circular object on a stand, 2 feet in diameter and divided into 4 different-colored panes of glass: Green, Blue, Yellow and Red.

He turned on the light bulb behind it and the barn was doused in a red glow of light. Then he turned the glass wheel to green. He told us that he used the colors to keep the animals healthy.

10 years later, I had moved to California. I met a well known acupuncturist who had several rooms, each with a different-colored light bulb. When I asked him why, he explained that he used Color Therapy on his patients and that they had benefited from it.

With these experiences, I began incorporating Color Therapy into my healing practice and found it to be simple, effective and sensible. In my healing room today, I have four individually colored light bulbs. I use each according to my clients needs. As a healer, you can also channel colors to achieve the same results, as you will learn in the upcoming exercise. Here is the core information you need to get started.

Remember the brain responds to all stimuli and directly affects the body's responses to them.

The Properties for Color Therapy Healing

Red: Penetrating; hot; used for deep coldness and low circulation and for fatigue. Use for 20 minutes or less (any more than 20 minutes becomes agitating rather than balancing.)

Yellow: Energizing; warm; optimistic; used for low energy, depression and mental alertness. Use for 30 minutes or less for the same reason.

Green: Regeneration; cellular repair; calming; opening the heart chakra; in the physical realm, used for bodily injuries (muscle tears, broken bones etc.); in the emotional realm, used for grief and depression. Again, 30 minutes or less.

Blue: Calming; sedating; used for anxiety, body inflammations and meditation. Again, 30 minutes or less.

Note: During a healing, turn off fluorescent lights as they disturb the body's electrical system.

173

Color Therapy: Exercise

1. Find a partner and sit facing each other, knee to knee.

2. Have your partner place their hands comfortably in their lap, palms up.

3. Place your palms 1 foot above their palms and channel one color at a time for at least 2 minutes. Relax, breathe, let go and let God.

4. Channel Red, Yellow, Green, Blue, Violet then White, telling your partner which color you're sending. Do this 2 times with each color.

5. Disengage and rest for a few minutes. Compare your experiences: what you felt as the sender and what they felt as the receiver.

6. Now, position yourselves again facing each other and this time choose one of the 5 colors and send it to your partner's palms. Don't tell them which one. Ask them what color they sense and then try another color. Have fun with it. It takes time to become sensitized to vibrational differences.

7. Finally, switch. Now you receive and they give. Repeat steps 1-6.

Once again practice, practice, practice. Everyone is a snowflake. We are all unique. You and your partner may experience the differences of vibrations visually, intuitively or in physical sensation. Learn to trust yourself. Try to let go of expectation and effort. Let go of the mind. Relax your arms and keep breathing in a natural rhythm. Channeling energy is not effort. It is letting it happen naturally. It is a state where you both may bask in the energy.

Hands-on Healing with Color

A client comes to you for a healing after a car accident. She is weak and has broken her ankle. During whichever healing technique you have chosen, you can add a color frequency directly to her injured ankle to accelerate cell rejuvenation (Green).

If the ankle is still inflamed, you will need to alternate Blue with Green, for a more effective healing.

Simply place one palm over the ankle and the other palm under it while drawing in the colors. You can incorporate this **localized color healing** into the general healing format at any time throughout the session.

Note: Start off with the color but then allow the color to change on its own. The client's energy system may automatically draw in a more needed color vibration.

Localized Polarity

Now that you have some knowledge of Color Therapy, the next step is to combine Color Therapy with the Polarity Healing technique.

Using the negative and positive poles of the palms, couple your palms around the affected area, such as a shoulder or knee. Let's use the knee as an example. One palm lays on the *front* of the knee and the other palm holds the *back* of the knee. Allow no less than five minutes for the circuit between the poles of your palms to connect and charge the knee. An alternate version would be to place your palms on each side of the knee.

If the knee is inflamed due to arthritis, bruised or has been burned, channel in the color Blue to sedate the inflammation. If the knee is cut or broken, use Green to regenerate cellular production.

With major organs, such as the liver or stomach, do the same; one palm on the front and one on the back of the body. The idea here is to surround the affected area to enable more complete healing by energy penetrating through it. Livers are often hot (high levels of energy when out of balance), so alternating blue and green energy is very effective.

Kidneys, on the other hand, tend to be cold or have a low level of energy. If this is the case, use Red and Yellow to energize this organ.

Caution: Do not use Green when dealing with arthritis and cancers in your clients. These diseases are caused by an overproduction of cells. Since Green *increases* cellular production, it would only aid the disease, not relieve it.

Finally, whenever in doubt, simply channel White, Violet or Reiki energy.

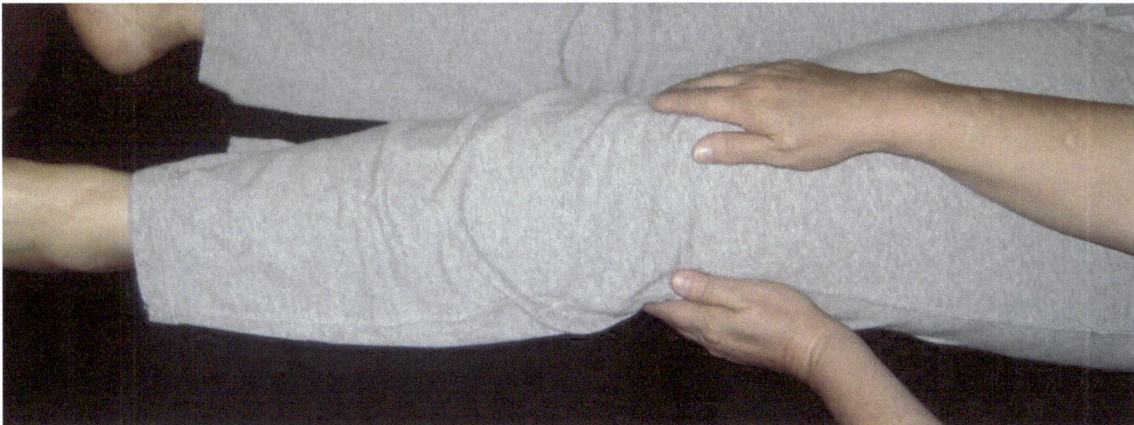

This healer is channeling blue on the client's knee.

Polarity Balancing with Color Imagery
(Polarity Technique while channeling and verbalizing each chakra color)

A good healer is also an educator. I like to teach my clients as I work on them if they're open to it. Sometimes during a Polarity healing, I will channel in each color to the corresponding chakra verbally so that the client can participate in the healing by focusing on it.

Occasionally, this can be tiring for them. At those times, it is not appropriate. Therefore, before you begin a healing, ask your client if they want to participate in some imagery methods during their healing session.

Chakra Imagery for the Client

Begin the Polarity Balance healing. As you reach each chakra, quietly guide them with this imagery:

Crown: "Imagine seeing a beautiful white light radiating out from the crown of your head. Breathe it in, let it expand all around you as you merge with spirit."

Third Eye: "Imagine now a deep purple light shining out from your forehead eliciting intuition and clarity."

Throat: "See a sky-blue color emanating from your throat and enveloping your neck and shoulders. Breathe in and let it expand for your sense of freedom and expression."

Heart: "Now, breathe in emerald green into your heart and let it fill you and expand all throughout your chest and back with love, healing and compassion."

Solar Plexus: "Feel the color of the sunlight in your stomach. Breathe in its warmth and comfort and strength."

Sacral: "Now, breathe in the orange color of a campfire in this power area of confidence and vitality. Let it fill the organs and lower back."

Root: "Imagine now the red warm color of fire at the bottom of your spine, filling you with health, stability and capability."

Remember to allow the client to rest between each chakra imagery. After you have guided them through the chakra totem, suggest that they relax their mind as you continue their healing in silence. This technique is very empowering for most clients and a valuable tool for them to practice at home.

Allowing your clients to participate actively in their own healing assists in the healing process itself. There is a mind-to-body connection being made. The mind says "Yes, I will help." and the body follows the mind's lead in promoting faster recovery and a sense of overall well-being. The healing is not an act being done to them. It is a combined effort between the healer's guidance and the intention of the client to heal.

A Client's Vision

You don't always want to manipulate or force color in a healing. The client's body/mind co-consciousness knows what it needs, often more than you do as the healer.

Example: I was guiding this color imagery with a client and noticed that he was agitated during the process. I quieted myself and intuited something was "off". I waited patiently and meditatively for my own guidance. I finally had the "knowing" and asked him, "What color are you seeing?" he answered, "Blue." I then guided him to bask in the blue and relax. His body needed that one color vibration for balance. I proceeded with and completed the healing session without any further interruptions. Healing begins as a skill and develops into an art.

Magnetic Polarity Technique (MPT): Introduction

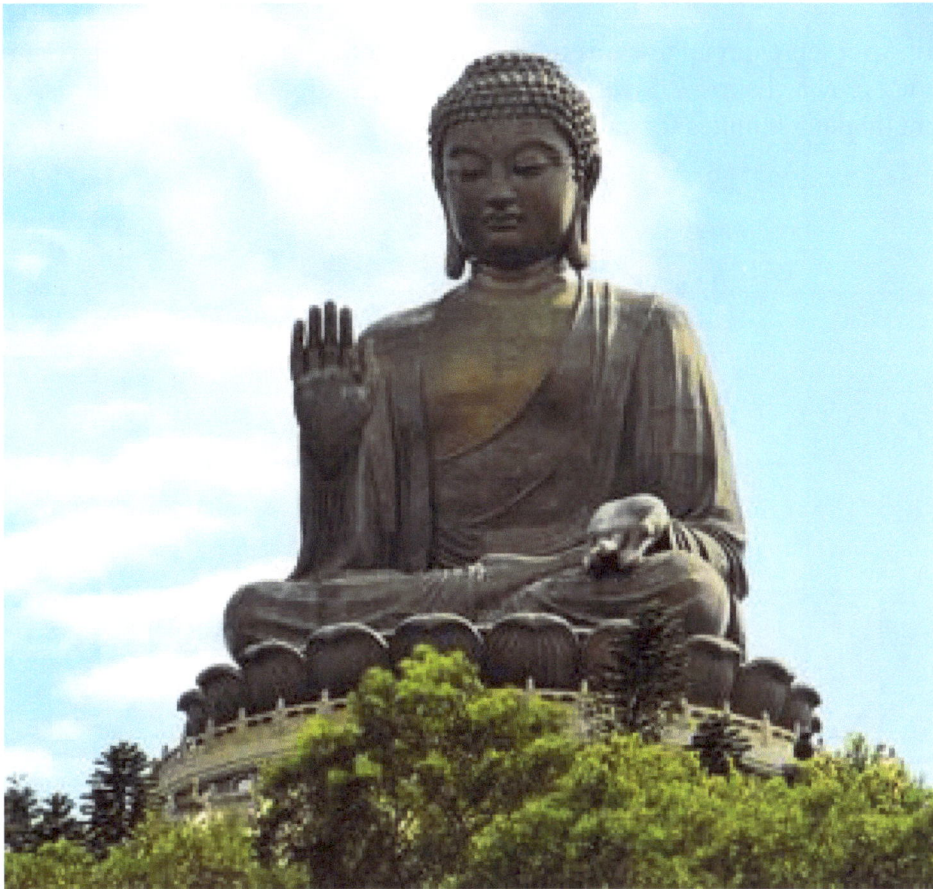

  Magnetic Polarity Technique, or MPT, is very simple. You will recall that our left hand "receives" and the right hand "sends". We are utilizing the negative and positive poles of magnetism.

  You may have seen Buddha statues like the one pictured above. As you can see, in the position he is depicted as assuming, he is sitting with his left hand on his lap with palm facing up to the sky (*receiving* life chi force) while his right palm is also up but facing out to the world (*sending* chi). This is magnetic polarity healing. The next few pages will detail the instructions and tips for this technique.

Magnetic Polarity Technique

1. Prepare yourself and the healing environment as usual.

2. Position your left palm up towards the North magnetic pole and place your right palm over your client's crown chakra. Allow time for the energy to flow like a stream from above to your client (about 5 minutes for each chakra).

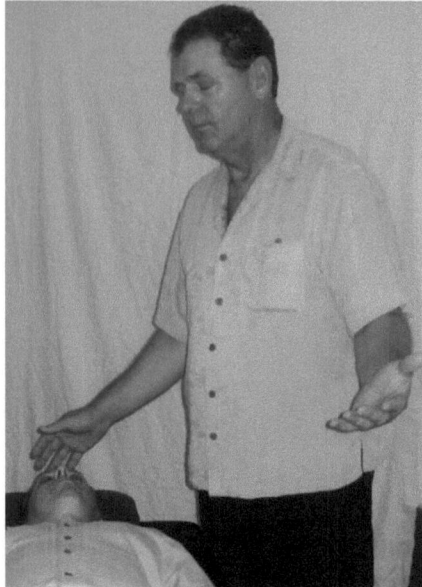

Example of using Magnetic Polarity at the crown chakra

3. Continue in the same procedure for each chakra (Third eye, throat, heart etc.). While doing this, your left palm is always facing to the sky or north (you can sit and rest your hand on your lap), while your right palm sends chi to the chakras.

Removing blocks along the way

4. While you are moving from chakra to chakra, if you feel a blockage in any chakra, do the following: Use your right hand and spin the chakra counter-clockwise, as if scooping out the blockage and pulling it out and tossing it towards the earth to release it. Repeat as many times as you feel is required. It is *imperative* to refill that chi energy before moving onto the next chakra by sending (with your right hand) chi back into that chakra.

You may also feel blocked energy on your hands. It may feel as if they're dirty or heavy. To clear this away, periodically shake it off your hands towards the ground in a downward motion away from your client. This will insure that you do not carry it with you after the healing.

5. It is that simple. After the healing, sweep and bubble as usual.

The MPT Vibration

This vibration is enhanced even more when placing the appropriate stones on the client's body at each chakra point and surrounding the table with a quality crystal vortex. I will introduce you to stone healings in a later chapter.

MPT and Infections

MPT is excellent for infections. I've used it dozens of times and it has always proven to be successful. You can also use it for sinus blockages, inflammations and overall energizing for a client. Also, remember you can guide the client with the chakra color imagery while you are moving to each chakra or just channel the chakra colors yourself.

Caution

If a client has a localized infection (as was the case with my client Lisa's story), never massage or touch the body surrounding the infection. By doing so, you could spread the infection. In these situations, work *only* in their auric field.

Alternate Hand Positions to Remove Stubborn Blocks

1. Place your left/receiving hand over the blocked area.
2. Your right/sending hand faces down to the earth.
3. After removing block, refill the area as before with right/sending chi and left hand facing up.

Long Distance and Group Healings
Energy follows thought

Long distance healing is a common practice in many cultures and ours is no different. You may have already practiced this in a general way. Have you ever heard someone relay an illness of a relative who lives miles away and say, "I'll keep them in our prayers". Prayer, too, is a form of healing. It is sending positive energy to a specific person or situation.

Almost every technique outlined in this book may be used for long distance healing. Below are the basic instructions. When in doubt, just send a simple prayer of hope, strength and thoughts of well-being.

Preparation:

1. Always ask for permission to do a healing whenever possible. Otherwise just send prayerful love that "They be given whatever is best and right for them at this time".

2. Always do your own chakra imagery before a healing. Smudge yourself and focus on your healing/spiritual mind set and altar. You may also hold a crystal specifically chosen for healing work if you want. Quartz crystals, for example, not only energize but boost transmissions of energy whether it's in the same room or across the miles.

Methods:

1. Place a piece of paper with the person's name on it between your palms. Ask their angel guides to join in sending the healing to them. Simply be in a prayerful/meditative state as you see their name written in the universe and as you send the healing rays to their name. Afterwards, place the paper on your altar or in a God Box, (which you will find in Volume 2 of the Healing Arts Series) for as long as you wish. Do this 2 or 3 times a day for at least 3 days consecutively.

2. Imagine the person's body in front of you and literally do a healing on the imagined body from start to finish. After this healing, follow up with Method number 1.

3. Use a doll or stuffed animal to represent the client for the healing and again follow up with method number one. You can perform this or other healing methods with a group as well.

Group Healings

Guidelines:

1. No more than 3 people should do a healing on a client. More than 3 may energetically "overload" the person, resulting in a negative rather than positive affect. Keep it simple.

2. The healers should be of compatible vibrations. When healing in a group, it is essential that all parties are agreeable. You want the highest, most positive vibrations working here without disagreements or misunderstandings on when or how to do the healing.

Group healing is an art. The goal of the healers is in creating a flowing, in-sync dance-like treatment. Choose one healer to lead the process from start to finish.

What is Reiki?

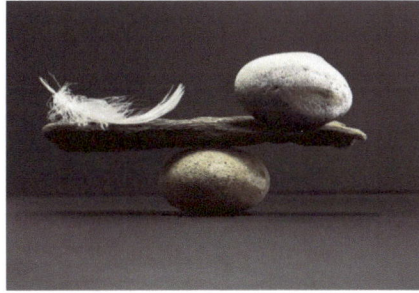

Reiki has become a popular healing technique in America and that's the good news. However, I am concerned about who is teaching it and how it is being taught. So, here are my thoughts.

If you're looking into taking the courses, I suggest you do a little research.

1. **Who is the teacher?** Ask the teacher how long they have been a healer; how many classes they have taught and if they practice any other healing techniques.

In my experience, the more techniques a person knows, the better a teacher they are. Practicing different methods educates a healer to the subtle yet significant differences in the frequencies and vibrations of the energies interacting between the client's energy body and the specific healing method (energy grid) being used. This, therefore is the teacher who knows the difference with the Reiki vibration and can incorporate elements of other techniques when needed. Reiki is not just a technique. It is the white light-higher, more energetic, even holy, if you will- and sometimes will bounce off the body because of density of physical or emotional obstacles. An experienced healer realizes this and can use other methods to shift the blocks and help Reiki flow in.

2. **How is it taught**? I highly advise you to attend classes that are 6 weeks or longer, unless you are already a healer.

The 3-day classes that are often offered may be inspiring and awakening to healing work but consider it only as an introduction to the healing art. I teach a 6 to 8-week course for each of the 3 levels for Reiki certification. Throughout the decades many of my students attended my course after having taken the weekend courses elsewhere, stating that they didn't feel like they knew what they were doing. In my courses, I teach them other techniques first (those in this manual), then Reiki. And, Yes, they knew, felt and saw the difference in energetic vibrations. It's a wonderful experience for them and I to see their growth within a mere 20 weeks.

3. **Becoming a Master**. Although I am certified as a Reiki Master, I find that position an insult to the true meaning of the word. No one is a Master in a weekend or a 20-week course. But that is another book to be written.

Lastly, again I am truly relieved, hopeful and gladdened that our western culture is discovering, exploring and embracing Reiki and other holistic health remedies. So, let's take the baton and pass it on. Keep going. Keep growing.

Test: Healing Techniques
(For Certification)

Requirements:

Please answer each question on a *separate sheet(s) of paper*. For certification purposes include the following:

- Your name
- Date you are completing this test
- Write/type out each question, then answer it.

20 Chakra Balancing

1. What pressure points do you press before this healing technique and why?

2. If you have your right palm on a client's ankle and your left palm on their knee, which hand moves next to the hip chakra?

3. How do you determine when it is time to move onto the next hand placement/chakra?

4. What conditions are best served by this technique?

Polarity Balancing Technique

1. How would you explain Polarity healing to a new client?

2. Which palm is the negative pole and what does that mean?

3. If the right hand is the positive pole, is it receiving or sending (projecting) energy?

4. Which palm would you place at the crown of a male client?

5. In every healing, you would channel energy on an area for no less than how many minutes?

6. If a client is having problems in the left side of their body, what might this imply?

Localized Polarity and Color

1. Describe this technique; how you place your hands and why?

2. What color would you channel for a broken bone?

3. What color would you channel for inflammation, such as a sprained ankle?

4. What color would you *not* use for cancerous growth?

5. Whenever in doubt, what color can you channel that is safe for all conditions?

6. What color sedates and relaxes?

7. What colors are energizing?

8. What is the difference between using red versus yellow for energizing?

9. What color elicits intuition and transformation?

Magnetic Polarity Technique (MPT)

1. Explain how to do this technique.
2. This technique is most beneficial for what conditions?

Long Distance Healing

1. How does long distance healing work?
2. Which method do you prefer?
3. Do you have your own method/ idea? Describe it.
4. Reiki is a high vibrational healing frequency. Why is it beneficial to know a variety of healing techniques and or frequencies?

Group Healing

1. How do you synchronize an effective group healing?
2. Why could too many healers in a group healing result in an in-effective healing? (thought question)

Chapter 7

The Shaman Path
Healing with Crystals and Stones

"Every part of this earth is sacred to my people. Every shining pine needle, every sandy shore, every mist in the dark woods, every clearing and every humming insect is holy... we are part of the earth and it is part of us... we all belong to the same family."

CHIEF SEATTLE TO THE US PRESIDENT IN 1854

Stone Healing: Introduction

Why use Stone Healing?

In the world we live in today, we are simply out of touch with nature. Using stones to heal helps us to instill a deeper connection or re-connection with nature and reminds us of the guidance and support that surrounds us always. Shaman healers often use stones.

Stones, Gems and Quartz all carry their own unique energy signature. Every one of them has energy to offer that is uniquely their own.

All stones are made up of minerals and each one of those minerals can be found in the human body. From the carbon in quartz crystals to the sodium in Sodalite, we share these properties with them. Doesn't it make sense, then, that stones can aid in healing?

I must admit, I'm partial to stones. I'm one of those people who likes to play in the mud, explore caves, hike in the mountains and climb over boulders. It's rare that I don't have a stone or pebble in my pocket or set in jewelry. I am amazed at how many stones there are and in what sizes, shapes, designs and colors they come. They are blossoms like any other.

How to connect with Stone Energy

The next time you notice a stone or rock on the ground, take some time and study it. Is it round, oblong, heart shaped, square? Does it have sharp edges? Is it colorful? Does it have cracks that map out like a spider's web or is it solid? Smooth or rough? Does it remind you of a boot, or wheel, or some other shape?

A stone is a wonderful meditation tool, one that you can do with your eyes open. It is like focusing on a candle flame. Concentrate on it. Let your mind wander with it and see what comes up.

I offer Shaman Stone readings based on the Medicine Wheel (more on this subject and on the Shaman Path in Volume 2). Unlike Tarot readings, the client assists in interpreting the stones. Stone readings are very revealing because they mirror one's inner nature.

Using stones to contribute to a healing is like adding a battery booster to it. Stones are a great tool to enhance the energy flow, remove blockages and adds an earth element to a general healing. There are several stones listed below, correlating to each chakra for balancing and healing. Next to each stone are its basic properties. Depending on what resource you use, you may find different stones to use for each chakra with additional properties. The study of shamanism is one of the best resources for understanding stone healing. Experiment on yourself and others and find what works best for you.

And know, not every healing needs to be done with stones. It is yet another option in the vast realm of healing techniques available to us as practitioners of the Healing Arts.

For a list of alternative and additional stones, see page 201.

In Volume 2 of this series, *Traveling the Wyrd Path* by Julie Bradshaw, there are several more in-depth and unique quartz and stone layouts to work with including another list of additional stones to use. If you are a stone lover, as well as a shaman path walker, you will love this book.

Stones for Chakra Balancing & Healing

All stones can be placed on the body or under the healing table at each chakra location.

Chakra	Stone	Energy Properties	Physical / Healing Properties	Placement
Crown	Rose Quartz	Promotes inspiration, attunes to divine love, protects the aura, unites dualities	Clears out cellular toxins, diminishes pain and stress, promotes serenity	Top of head
3rd Eye	Amethyst	Develops intuition, insight, promotes peace, clarity and meditation	Balances the endocrine and nervous system, relieves insomnia, headaches eye and ear disorders	Center of forehead
Throat	Lapis	Promotes self-expression, courage, creativity, protects the aura, unites dualities	Relieves insomnia, vertigo, hearing loss, supports the immune system	On top of the Throat
Heart	Malachite	Facilitates insight to the causes of body/mind/spirit conditions, unifies human/divine love	Enhances the immune system for overall healing and wellness	On top of the Heart
Solar	Citrine	Relieves anger, fear, depression, promotes self-worth, confidence and achievement	Relieves digestive ailments, cleanses the blood, improves all systems of the body	On top of the stomach
Sacral	Carnelian	Restores physical energy, releases apathy and addictions, promotes self-trust, heals emotional traumas	Relieves neuralgia, gall/kidney, allergies, spine, spleen, pancreas, sexual disorders	Below the bellybutton
Root	Red Jasper	Strengthens physical, mental, emotional, spiritual bodies, grounds, focuses, directs to manifest goals	Fosters physical strength, vitality, endurance, balances minerals for organ health	Just below where the thighs meet

Charging the stones

Each stone will need to be charged before a healing. You can simply lay them out in the sun or on the earth for a few hours. Occasionally, lay all your stones on the earth for at least 24 hours. They need the nourishment from nature just as we do.

Cleansing the stones before and after healing

Cleansing is also important to rid the stones of any negative or static energy they may have picked up along the way. You can wash them in a bowl of water mixed with rock or sea salt. Smudge your stones as well, much like you would smudge yourself or your client before and after a healing. Use sage, cedar or pine.

Stone Healing Technique

1.   Begin by performing the healing procedure on page 140

2.   Have your client lie flat on the floor or on a massage table. Place the stones on the client's body, as shown in the following diagram. It helps to use a cloth or small piece of felt in the correlating colors to keep the stones from falling off. You can also use strings of stone chips.

3.   Start at the root chakra, placing your palms just a few inches above the stone. Channel Chi into the stone, releasing the stone's energies in accordance with it's properties.

4.   Repeat this step over each chakra.
As with many of the other techniques you will use, you may feel a temperature change or tingling in your hands. Take as much time as needed to balance each chakra with the stone energy. *The Magnetic Polarity Technique is also a good choice to use.*

5.   When you've finished at the crown chakra, give your client a few minutes to just lie with the stones still in place. This would be a great time to add *sound frequency*. It's a glorious experience!

6.   When it's time to end the healing, gently remove the stones from your client, starting with the crown chakra. The piece of felt or cloth makes it easier to retrieve them. Set the stones aside for cleansing later. Then, sweep and bubble as usual.

Closing:
Give them a few more moments and gently bring them out of the healing space, like bringing them out of meditation. Guide them to become aware of their physical body and surroundings. And then finally to open their eyes.

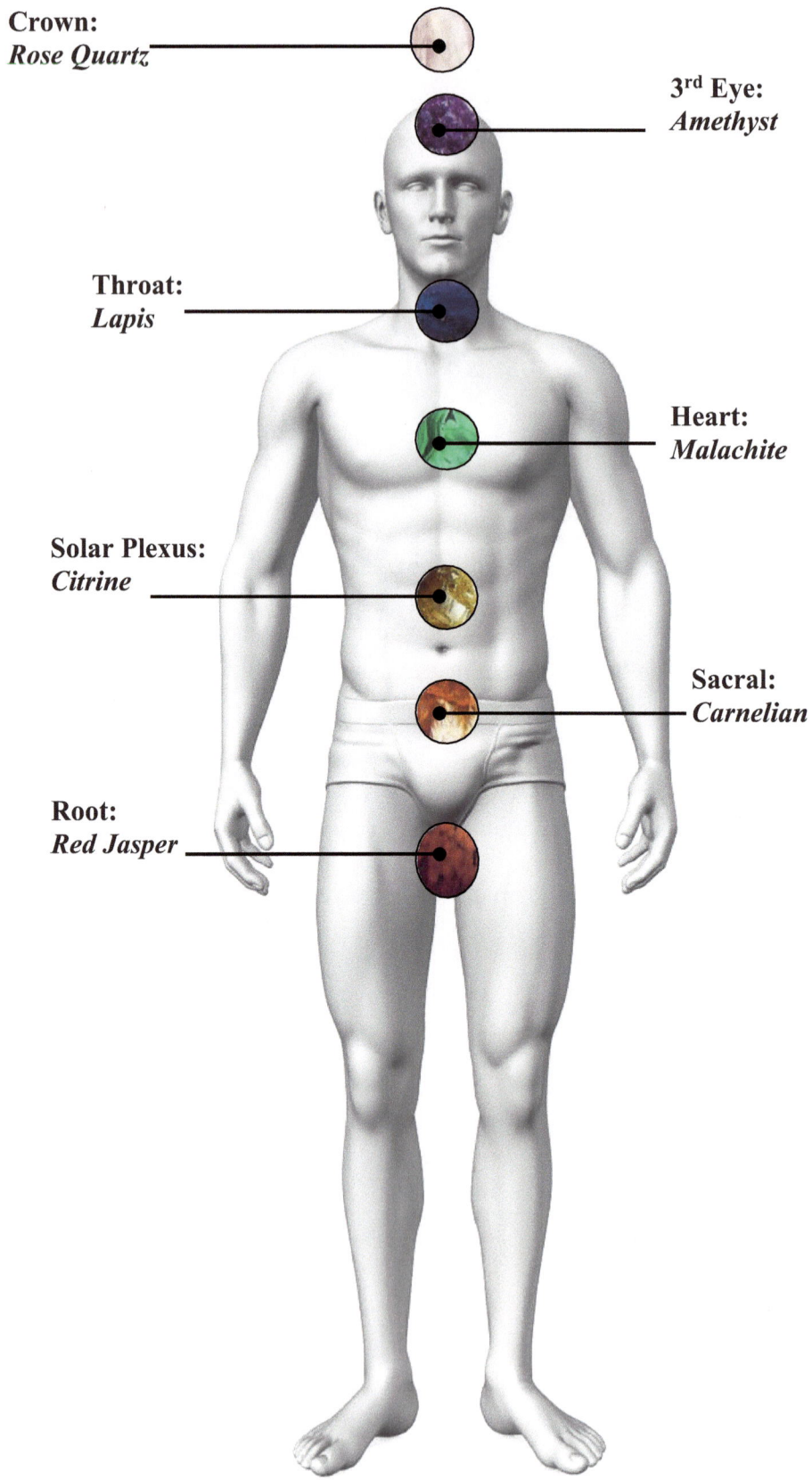

Crown:
Rose Quartz

3rd Eye:
Amethyst

Throat:
Lapis

Heart:
Malachite

Solar Plexus:
Citrine

Sacral:
Carnelian

Root:
Red Jasper

Quartz Crystal Healing Layouts: Introduction

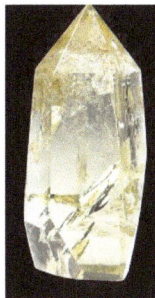

Single Terminated Natural

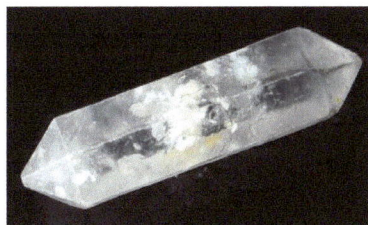

Double Terminated Natural

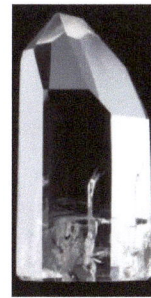

Single Terminated Polished

When it comes to crystals, Quartz crystal is probably the most recognizable. It has been associated with the "New Age" movement which started around the 1960's and has continued to gain notoriety through to present day. What most people don't realize is that quartz crystal is also used in the making of watches, telephones, clocks and much more.

Quartz crystal is a conductor of and storage unit for, energy. That is why it's so popular with healers and scientists alike.

How and why they work

Quartz crystals were created in the earth through pressure and temperature. They embody a unique arrangement of atoms, molecules and ions forming a crystalline six-point structure. They are composed of a pattern and lattice, exhibiting long range order and symmetry. Because of this unique structure they have electrical properties which, when sourced, emit an electrical pulse of precisely defined accuracy. This is why quartz crystals have been used for radios, clocks and watches. When sourced by pressure or movement, they ensure accuracy.

In using them for healing purposes, the source comes from nature and a conduit of energy.

Acutrigger Healing Tool

Quartz crystals need a source to stimulate the electrical particles. There is a tool called an "Acutrigger" I recommend. You can find it online. It replaces the original Acuspark, which is no longer available. It is a device containing a quartz crystal that is activated when you push the button. Inside the chamber, a hammer strikes the crystal, producing a *piezoelectric* (pressure sourced) energy pulse. I use this on acupressure points on the body, **as well as on each base of the crystals along the layout**.

What crystals to use?

For the following techniques, use large, single terminated clear quartz crystal points. Just as in stone healing, you are using them as a tool to facilitate healing. Follow the same instructions for charging and cleansing.

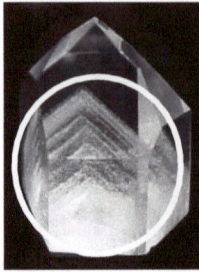

Phantom

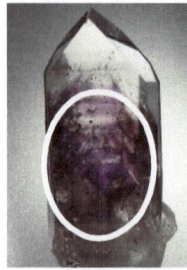

Amethyst
Inclusion

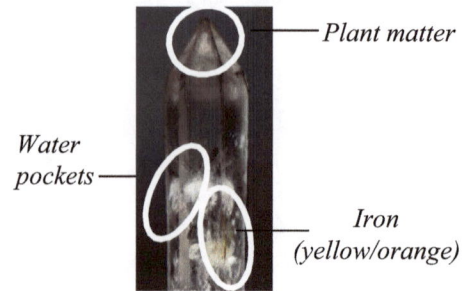

Water pocket plant &
iron inclusions

Plant matter

Water pockets

Iron (yellow/orange)

Some crystals may carry "inclusions ". These are bits of organic and inorganic material that were in the earth as the crystal grew. They may include iron or other minerals, small plants, other crystals or even water and air bubbles. (These last two are called "phantom"). This happens when a quartz crystal begins to grow, then stops and another crystal grows around it. It gives the appearance of two or more crystals in one, the first usually being slightly smaller and more opaque than the other. Try to purchase the clearest quartz available.

When performing a healing, ask the crystals for their assistance. State your goal or intention and thank them, before and after the healing. In essence, you are thanking Great Spirit who abides in them and all of life's healing properties.

My Native American and Celtic Shaman studies have taught me to ask and thank the earth for all it provides. In doing so, I have experienced a greater understanding that all of nature is alive with the same life force as ourselves. Just as we would, therefore, ask a friend for assistance and thank them for it, we do so with our herbs and stones as well.

It has been documented that when people talk to their plants, the plants thrive. Well, once again, energy follows thought.

The Techniques and Layouts

What is a Vortex?

Definition:

Vortex: *n.* **a whirling mass of something, especially water or air, that draws everything near it toward its center.**

In regard to energy, when you set a layout with crystals, it creates an *energy mass,* or *vortex,* which cycles and feeds itself. As a healer, you will be able to draw upon this concentrated energy to aid in healing a client or yourself.

It is imperative to learn how to use quartz properly. The crystals will intensify chaos or negativity, as well as order and your healing intention. Your intention in the healing must be clearly defined and the room, tools and all stones must be clean and clear of any disharmony.

Use these quartz crystal layouts without stones. Place the vortex under a chair or around you if you are lying down and relax for 15-30 minutes.

Healing Procedure For the Client

1) Cleanse the room.

2) Light the altar candle with a prayer of intention.

3) Discuss with your client their goals for this healing.

4) Place the vortex of crystals around a chair, on the table around your client or under the it and activate it using the Acutrigger or channeling red into each stone.

5) Perform the healing.

6) Remove the quartz crystals halfway through the healing.

7) Lastly, finalize the healing. Bubble your client and close the healing space then cleanse yourself, the room and the crystals.

Your Personal Healing

1) Use the Enlightenment vortex in the morning to gently wake up or heighten a meditation to start your day refreshed, clear and balanced.

2) Use the grounding vortex in the evening to destress and sleep soundly.

3) Use the Star of David when you need added energy or a 2nd wind in your life's routine.

This is only a suggestion. Since each of us is a unique individual, your response to each vortex may differ from others. So, use them as and when they suit you.

Grounding Vortex

For this technique, you will need three single terminated quartz points. When placing the crystals in this way, it creates a vortex of grounding energy.

Use this for stabilizing your clients in cases of anxiety, nervous conditions, and instability. It may also be used for bringing your wishes into the physical world, deep healing of the physical body and regaining strength after an illness.

Set the Quartz *with* the grain of the body, pointed towards the feet. Charge and place the vortex on or under the healing table around the client.

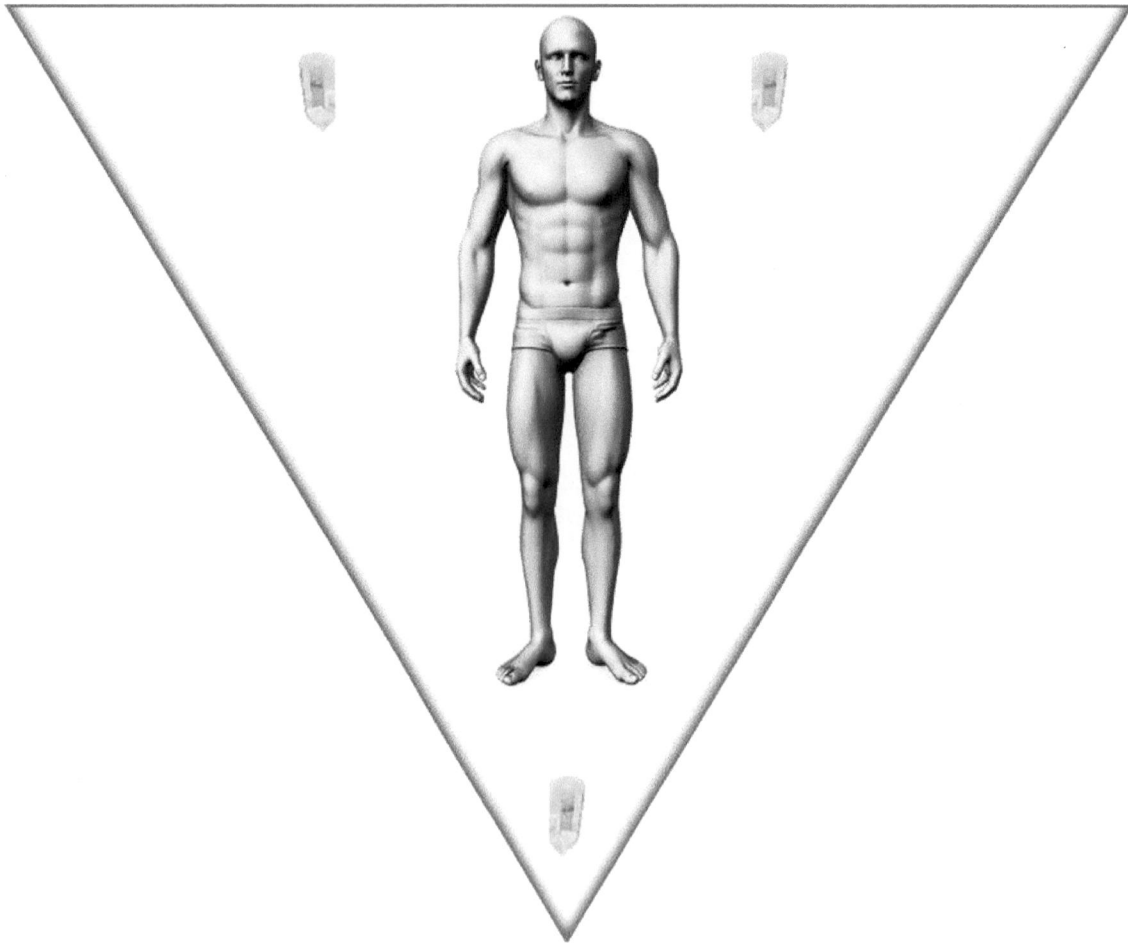

Enlightening Vortex

Lighten up!

The Enlightenment vortex is used primarily for meditation and connection with the Higher Self and the Divine. Use this layout when you feel stuck in a situation or if you're in a bad or lethargic mood. It may also be used for past life regression work. Only people in general good health should use this vortex. It is not recommended for small children, the chronically ill, the elderly or after major surgeries. Place and charge the upright triangle vortex on or under a healing table.

Set the Quartz *against* the grain of the body, pointed towards the head.

Important: After this vortex, use the "Grounding Vortex" on the previous page for five to ten minutes to re-establish their clockwise auric flow.

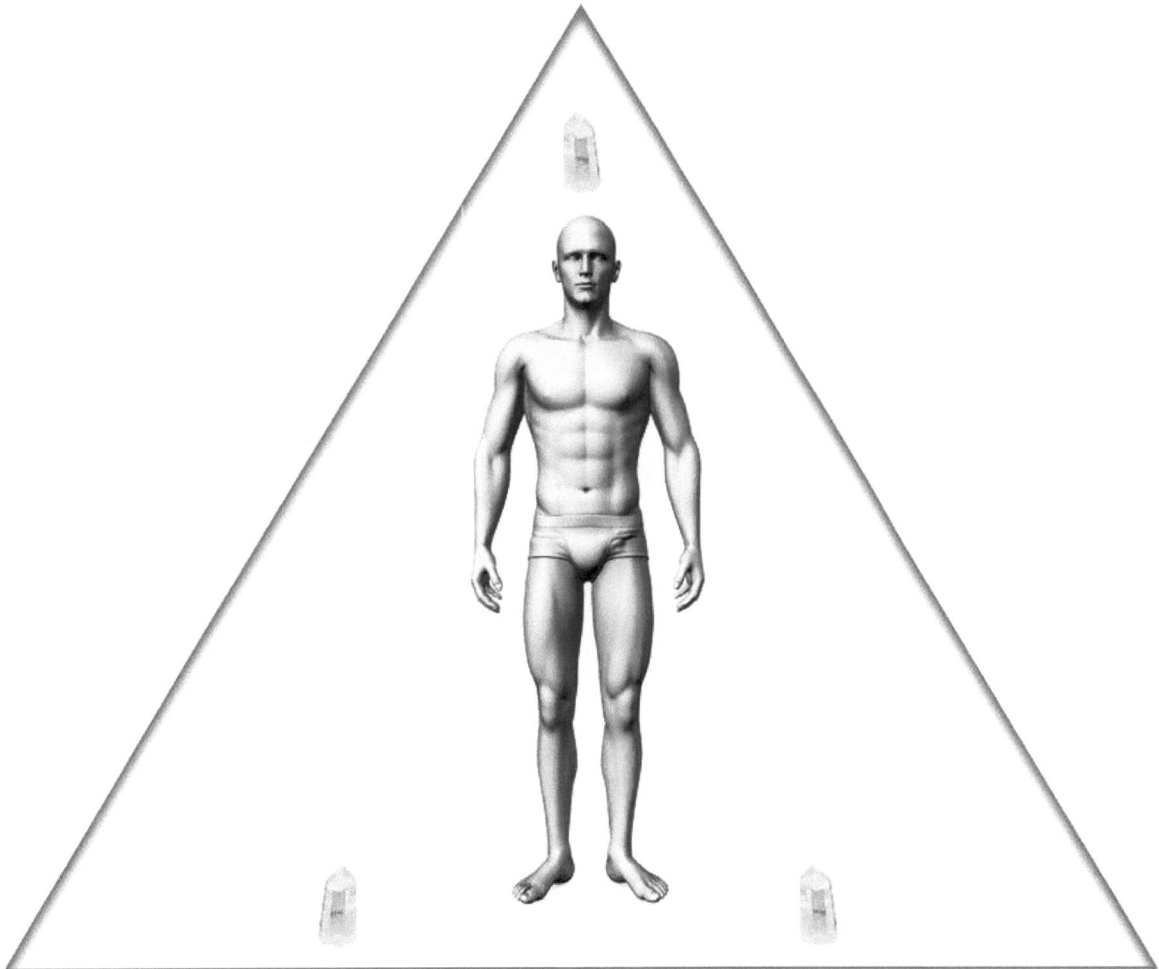

Star of David Vortex

This vortex combines the grounding and enlightening triangles. Use this layout to promote balance between opposite polarities and overall wellness. It can also help energize to combat fatigue. **Important:** double check that you've placed the points in the proper directions.

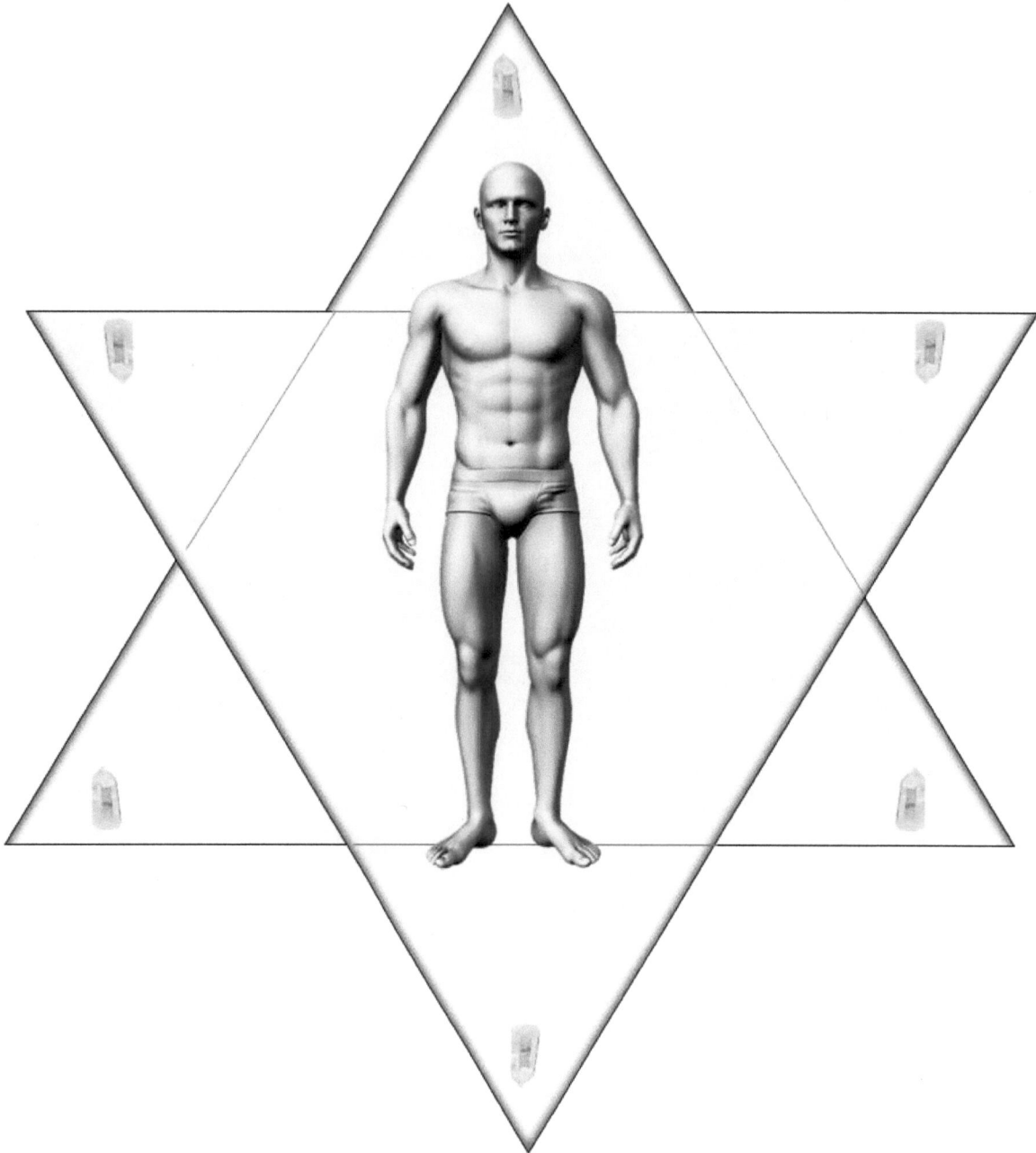

Quartz with Stone Layouts
for Aura Balancing

Ok, you've learned how to use the Chakra stones and the Quartz crystals for healing. Now it's time to put them together. The following pages show vortexes that use quartz crystals in conjunction with healing stones. By doing this, you will amplify the properties of the healing stones with the energy of the crystals, making them both stronger in their respective advantages.

Stone Properties

Like many of the healing techniques, you don't have to follow the rules laid out here to the letter to have a successful healing. Each client is different and what works for one may not work for another. Keep this in mind as you work with the stones and crystals. It may be that malachite works for one client's heart chakra while another may need rose quartz or turquoise. The combinations that can be used are limitless. Keep an open mind and listen to your intuition. Each stone has its own healing properties within its mineral content. A stone with Iron, for example, is a natural red blood cell enhancer.

The following layouts, which include healing stones, cleanse and balance the aura which is equally important as a Chakra balancing. Many healers focus solely on the primary Chakras not realizing that some debris can remain in the outer layers of the aura. An aura cleanse is immensely refreshing and the healing properties of the stones will expand out into the auric layers more readily due to the quartz vortex.

Grounding Vortex
(with stones)

For this technique you will need three single terminated quartz points with Amethyst, Rose Quartz and Jasper stones. This amplifies the vortex of grounding energy.

Use this for stabilizing in cases of anxiety, nervous conditions and instability. It may also be used for manifesting ideas into the physical world, deep healing of the physical body and regaining strength after an illness.

Set the quartz stones *with* the grain of the body, pointed towards the feet. Place the stones at each quartz point. Charge the vortex.

Properties of stones
Amethyst: Insight, intuition, meditation.
Rose Quartz: Peace, faith and union.
Jasper: Stability, strength and grounding.

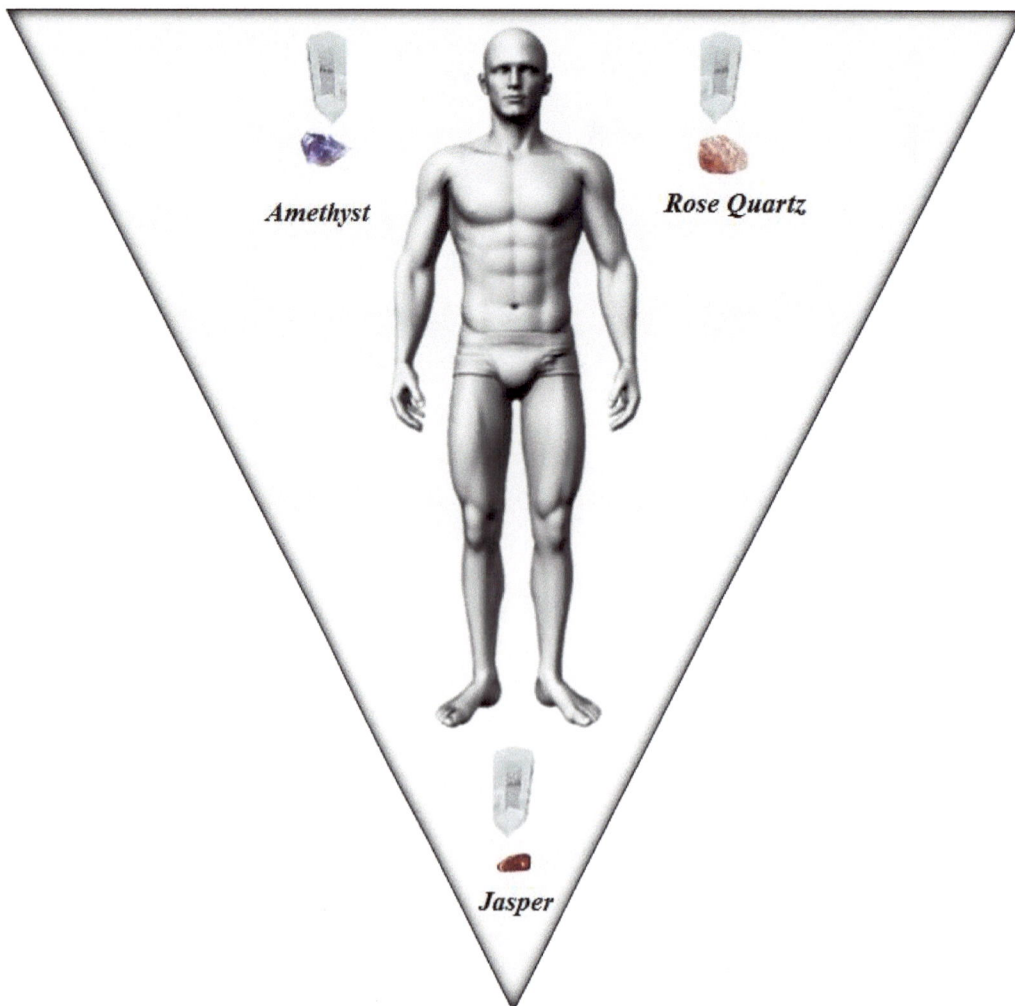

Amethyst

Rose Quartz

Jasper

Enlightening Vortex
(with stones)

Lighten up!

The Enlightenment vortex is used primarily for meditation and connection with the Higher Self and the Divine. Use this layout when you feel stuck in a situation or if you're in a bad or lethargic mood. It may also be used for past life regression work. Only people in general good health should use this vortex. It is not recommended for small children, chronically ill, elderly or after major surgeries.

Place the stones at each quartz point. Charge the vortex.

Properties of stones
Amethyst: Insight, intuition, meditation.
Rose Quartz: Peace, faith and union.
Citrine: Emotional healing, self-worth, inner strength and boundaries.

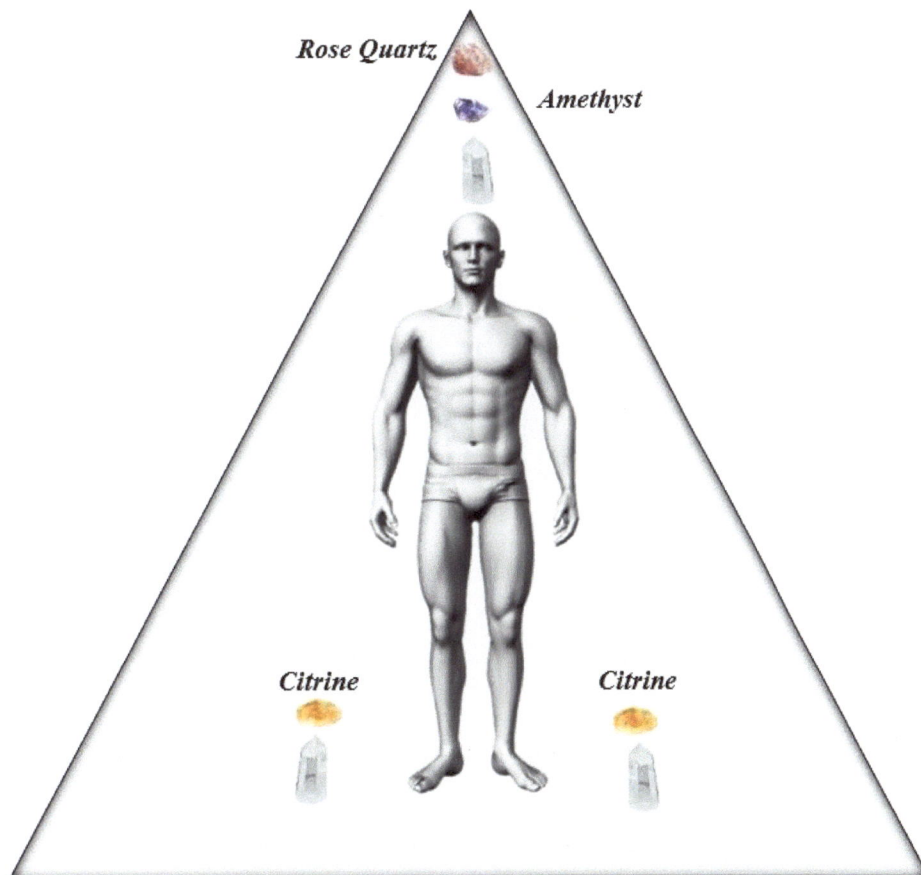

Star of David Vortex
(with stones)

Encompassing all

This vortex helps to unite the male and female, spiritual, physical aspects and promotes wholeness. It is an excellent layout for balance. It combines both the ground and enlightening vortexes.

You will use six crystals and six stones. The energies created in this vortex may stir up issues or blockages you may currently have, so it's great for breakthroughs. You may also add a Rose Quartz to the Heart Chakra. Double check proper placements of the quartz points.

Properties of stones

Amethyst: Insight, intuition, meditation.
Rose Quartz: Peace, faith and union.
Citrine: Emotional healing, self-worth, inner strength and boundaries.
Jasper: stability, strength and grounding

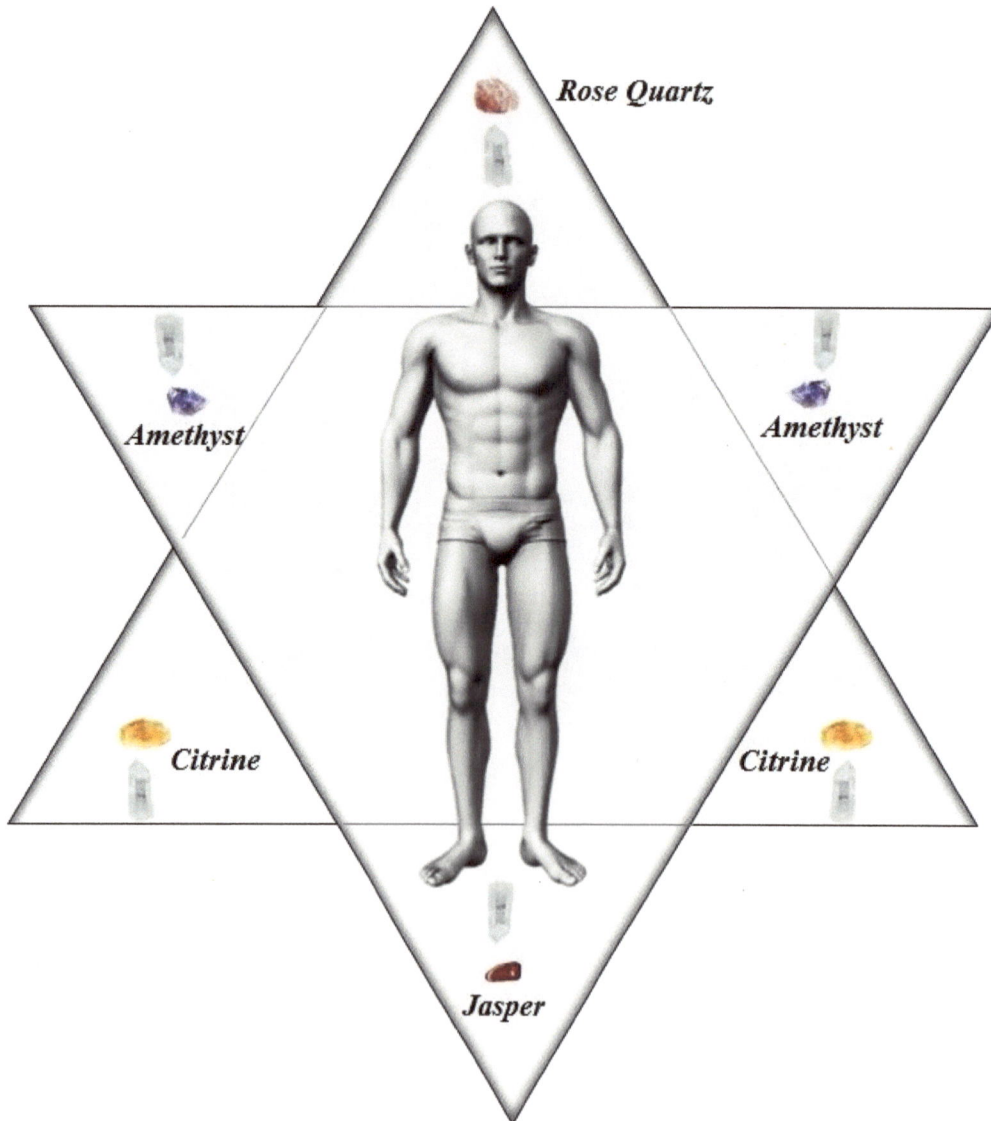

Rose Quartz

Amethyst

Amethyst

Citrine

Citrine

Jasper

Alternative and Additional Stones

As you work with stones, you will become more attuned with each of their vibrational healing properties. With this knowledge, you can choose which stone to use or add for your client's specific needs, especially regarding any glandular issues.

These additional stones can be added to the chakra stone layout, however, use no more than 3 stones on a chakra. But remember that more is not necessarily better.

Listen to your guidance and trust your intuition. Often times, simple and serene is more effective. I have had to learn this over and over again.

Note: If you're adding a Quartz crystal layout, remove all stone about halfway through the healing. It can be too stimulating otherwise in an hour's session.

Alternative Chakra Stones

Crown: *Rose,* Aurichalite for Pineal gland, Angel Wing Agate, Biotite Lens
3rd eye: *Amethyst*, Sillimanite for Pituitary gland, Tanzanite
Throat: *Lapis*, Betafite for Thyroid, Blue Coral, Blue Kyanite (upper chakra's cleanse)
Heart: *Malachite*, Chevron Amethyst for Thymus, Lepidolite
Solar Plexus: *Citrine*, Rose-Eye Agate for Pancreas, Bixbite, Apatite
Sacral: *Carnelian*, Hemimorphite for Gonads, pyrite
Root: *Red Jasper*, Chrysobery for adrenals, kidneys, onyx, garnet, ruby, Black Kyanite (lower chakra's blockage cleanse)

So, the above list of alternative stones are for the Chakra totem. The following list of stones can be added to the chakra totem or used by themselves in a vortex. Place the chosen stone on the affected chakra (ie: place the stone for stomach issues on the solar plexus).

Additional Stones

Addiction: Desert Rose, Dicinite, Lazulite
Allergies: Clevelandite, Cookeite, Muscovite
Anxiety: Azurite, Malachite, Black Sapphire
Constipation: Magnesioferrite, Fire Opal
Depression: Beudantite, Red Coral, Seamanite
Diarrhea: ILvaite, Okenite
Grief/Fear/Anger: Magnetite,Chlorite, Apache Tear, Onyx
Humor: Watermelon, Tourmaline, Wagnerite
Inner Self-awareness: Iris Agate, Waverllite, Alabaster
Insomnia: cookeite, Lepidolite, Rose
Instability: Magnesioferrite, Onyx, Red Jasper Petrified wood
Liver: Polka-Dot Agate, Yellow Sapphire
Maturity: Alabaster, Calomel, Alexandrite
Reiki: Zeolite, Mosandrite, Black or Green obsidian
Sexuality: Copper, Hummerite
Serenity: Amethyst, Bismuth, Rose
Toxins: Zeolite, Chlorite, Franckeite for mental release

Chapter 8

Healing with the Senses

"Our bodies communicate to us clearly and specifically,
if we are willing to listen to them."

SHAKTI GAWAIN

Reflexology

Reflexology is a holistic discipline, using the hands to apply pressure to the feet, hands, face and ears to stimulate the reflexes and nervous system of the body. There are hundreds of pressure points in the body that relate to each organ and energy system. Massaging these areas daily can reduce stress, increase circulation and balance the meridians. Happy feet, happy body!

Reflexology Points on the Face

The following diagrams are samples of acupressure points (accu-points). You can easily find detailed charts of accu-points via the internet if you are interested in further study.

I usually incorporate some points during a healing. Clients love it and I give them handouts to use at home.

Accu-points on the face may help relieve sinusitis, headaches, insomnia, anxiety and jaw tightness.

Massage and press each point for no less than 2 minutes each. Make sure to press points simultaneously (i.e. left and right side at the same time, as in the case of numbers 1 and 2 below). Refer to the diagram on the next page.

1. The top of the forehead.

2. The middle of the forehead.

3. Inside the eye socket (gently).

4. Pinch all along eyebrows.

5. Temples

6. Side of nostrils and following up under the cheekbones.

7. One finger deep inside the ear, pushing forward to unblock/stretch the jaw muscle.

8. Pinch from cheek muscle down to jaws.

9. Rub along the upper and lower teeth areas.

10. Press point below the nose and above the upper lip

11. Press point below upper lip and above chin.

12. Use three fingers to press chin firmly back to release the neck 3 times.

13. Tap the thymus gland located on the upper chest just above the heart chakra.

14. Have your client rotate their tongue to massage the inside of their mouth in one direction then the other.

This session should take at least 30 minutes. As a healer, you are still channeling a peaceful energy. After the session the client's entire body should feel balanced and rejuvenated as if they received a full body massage.

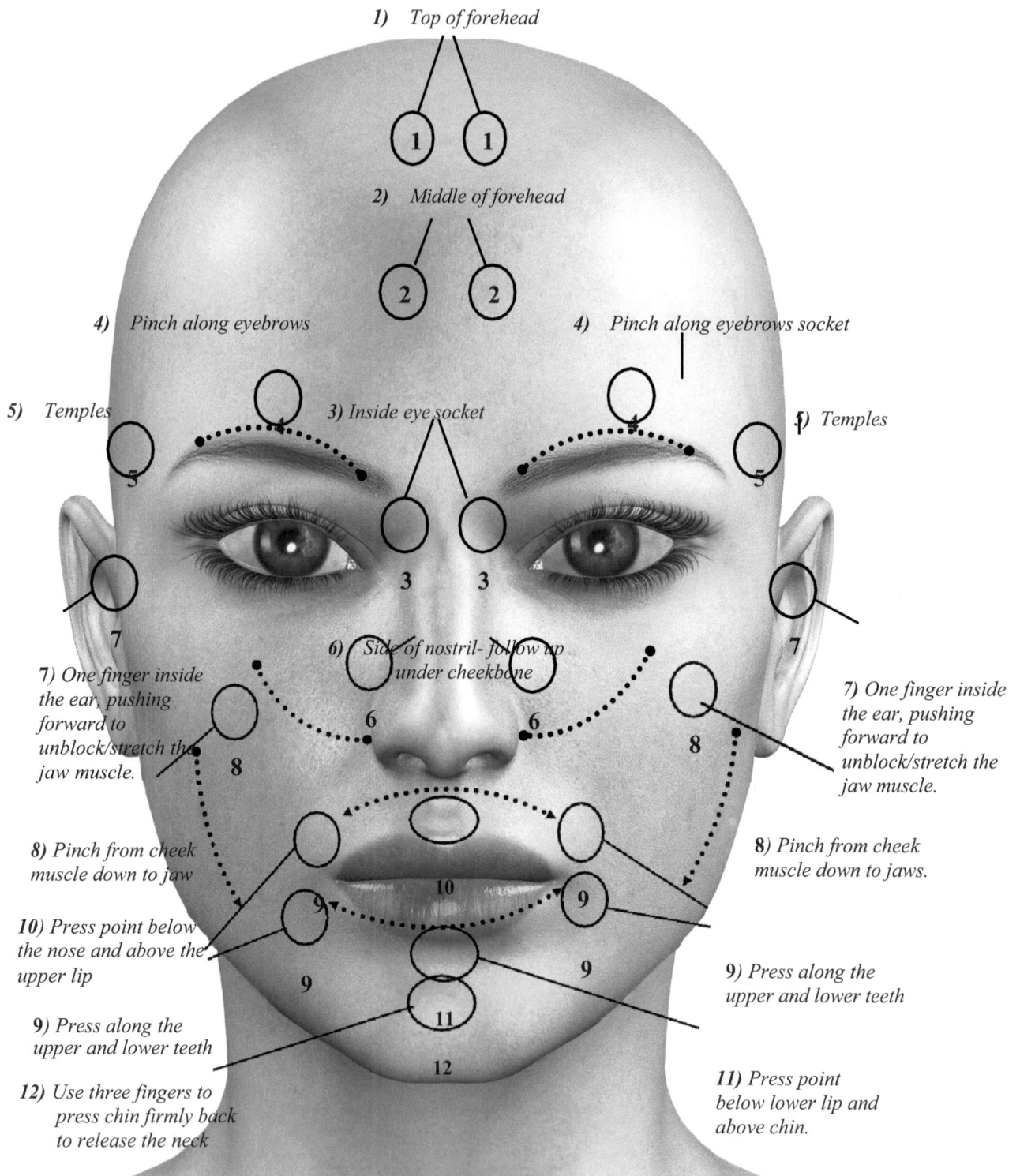

1) *Top of forehead*

1 1

2) *Middle of forehead*

2 2

4) *Pinch along eyebrows*

4) *Pinch along eyebrows socket*

5) *Temples*

3) *Inside eye socket*

5) *Temples*

6) *Side of nostril- follow up under cheekbone*

7) *One finger inside the ear, pushing forward to unblock/stretch the jaw muscle.*

7) *One finger inside the ear, pushing forward to unblock/stretch the jaw muscle.*

8) *Pinch from cheek muscle down to jaw*

8) *Pinch from cheek muscle down to jaws.*

10) *Press point below the nose and above the upper lip*

9) *Press along the upper and lower teeth*

9) *Press along the upper and lower teeth*

12) *Use three fingers to press chin firmly back to release the neck*

11) *Press point below lower lip and above chin.*

13) *Tap thymus gland (6 inches below the thyroid) 3 times*

14) *Lastly have your client rotate their tongue to massage the inside of their mouth in one direction then the other.*

206

Chakra Points on the Hands and Feet

Incorporate these acupressure points into a healing to aid in opening the chakras of the body. I like to begin every healing with this. It relaxes the clients, which makes it easier for them to receive the healing. It also makes clearing out blockages easier for me as the healer.

Hand Points

4) Massage the palm of the hands.
5) Massage the back of the hands.
6) Press and massage each point for about 2 minutes each.

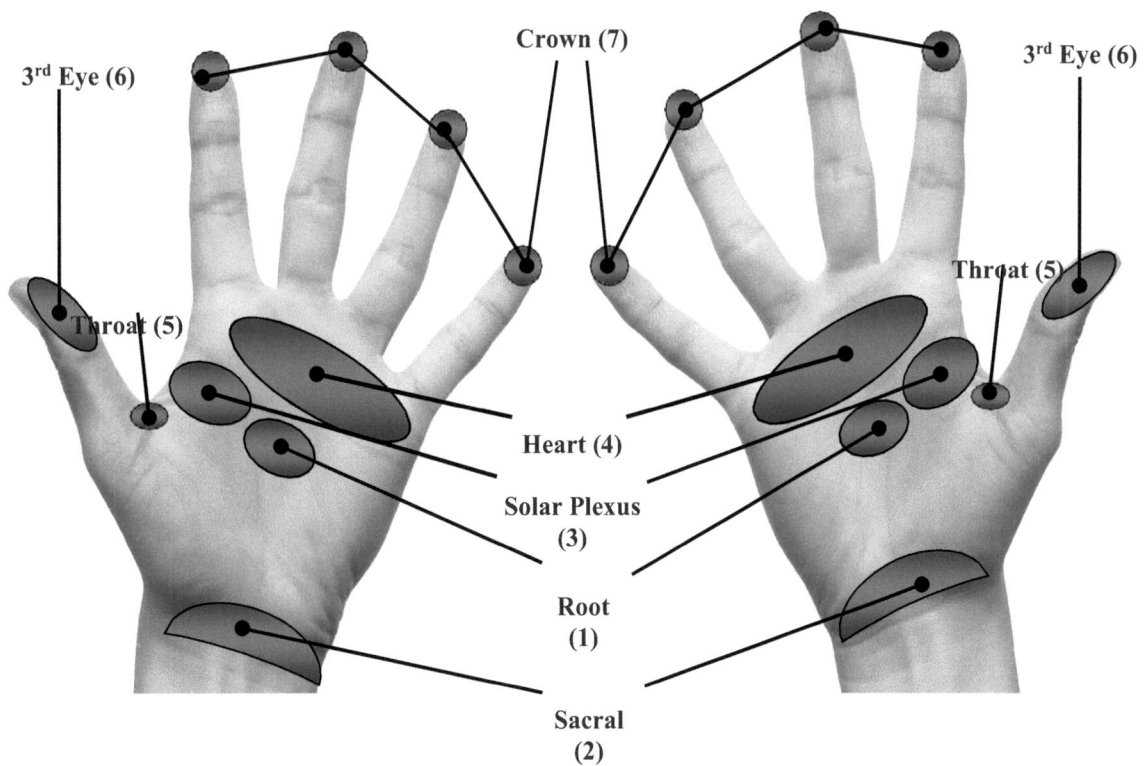

3rd Eye (6)

Crown (7)

3rd Eye (6)

Throat (5)

Throat (5)

Heart (4)

Solar Plexus (3)

Root (1)

Sacral (2)

Foot Points

Crown

3rd Eye

Throat

Heart

Solar Plexus

Root

Right Foot   **Left Foot**

Sacral / 2nd chakra

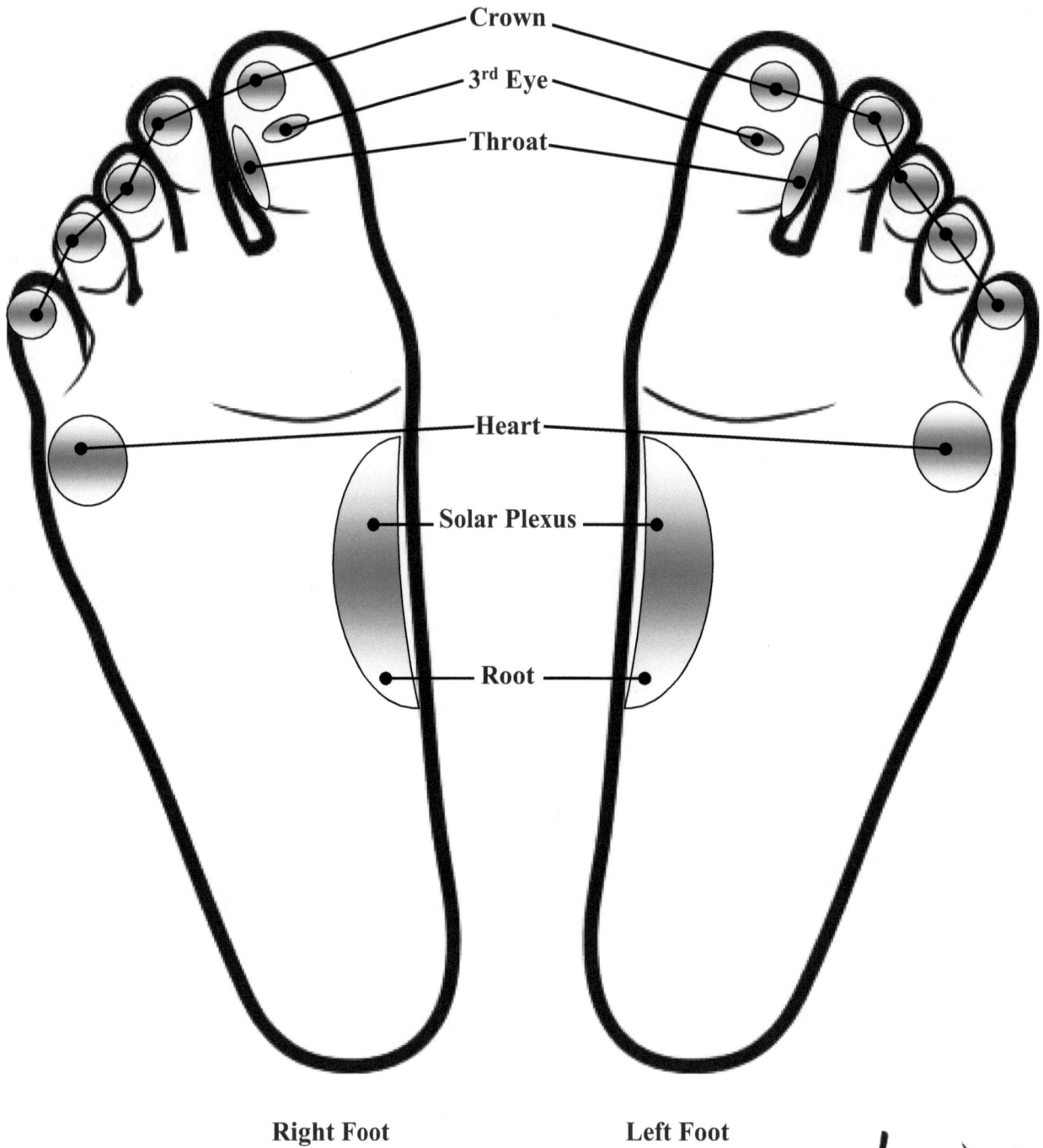

1. Massage up and down the entire sole of each foot.
2. Massage up and down the front (top) of each foot.
3. Press and massage each point simultaneously for not less than 2 minutes.

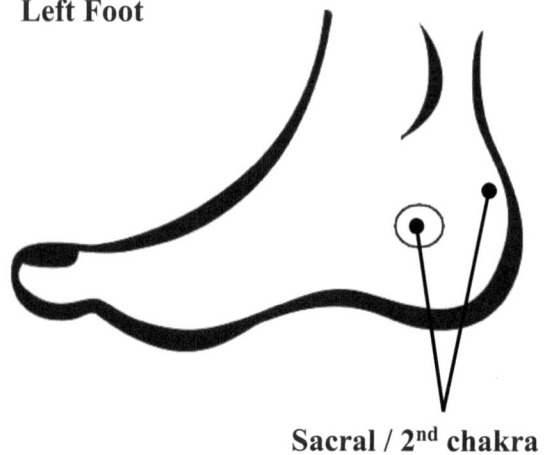

Acupressure Points for the Immune System

The following pressure points are adapted from Chinese Medicine. There are several hundred such points in the human body.

Meridian points are noted by a letter and a number. The letter denotes the area of the body. (For example: K = Kidney ST= Stomach). They are not all located on the organ itself but rather are related to the meridian of that organ. The number shows its exact location on the body.

The next few pages show the acupressure points on the front and back of the body and on the arm to aid in keeping the immune system running smoothly.

Press and massage these points for no less than 2 minutes each. You may simply incorporate them into the healing.

Elegant Mansion– (K 27)
Location: In the depression directly below the collarbone.
Benefits: Relieves chest congestion, breathing difficulties, asthma, coughing, anxiety and depression.

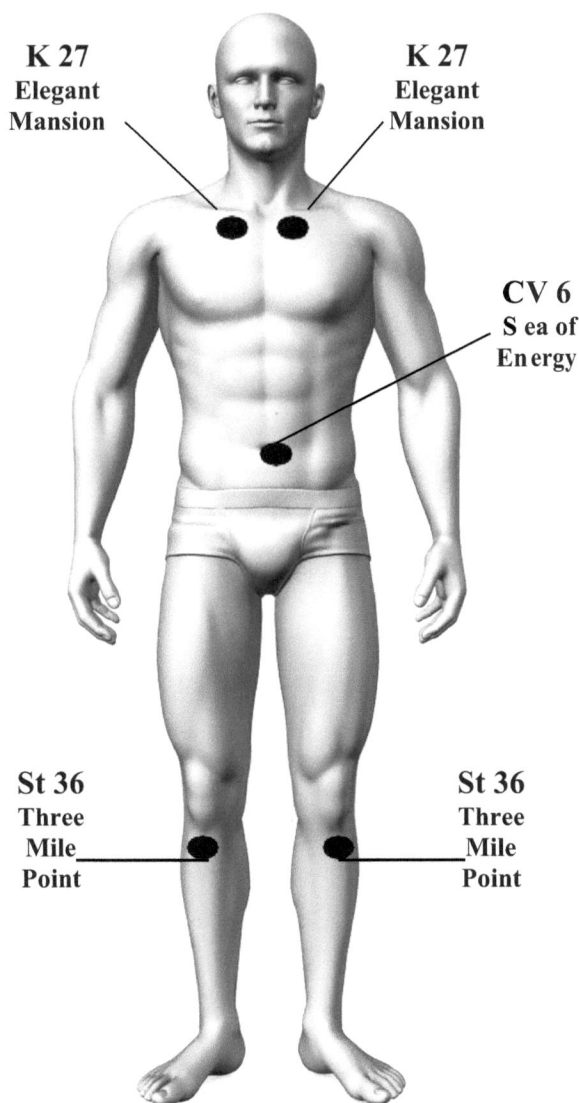

K 27
Elegant
Mansion

K 27
Elegant
Mansion

CV 6
S ea of
En ergy

St 36
Three
Mile
Point

St 36
Three
Mile
Point

Sea of Energy – (CV 6)
Location: Two fingers widths below the belly button.
Benefits: Relieves abdominal muscle pain, constipation, gas and general weakness.

Three Mile Point – (St 36)
Location: Four finger widths below the kneecap, one finger width to the outside of the shinbone.
Benefits: Strengthens the whole body, tones the muscles and aids digestion as well as relieves fatigue.
Important immune system point.

LI 11
Crooked Pond

Crooked Pond – (L 11)
Location: Upper edge of the elbow crease.
Benefits: Important immune system
point, relieves fever, constipation
and elbow pain.

LI 4
Joining the Valley (Hoku)

Joining the Valley (Hoku) – (LI 4)
Caution: not *for pregnant women because
its stimulation can cause premature
contractions in the uterus.*
Location: In the webbing between the thumb
and index finger.
Benefits: Relieves constipation, headaches,
toothaches, shoulder pain, labor pain, arthritis.

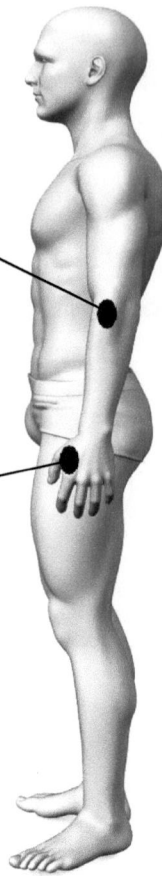

Sea of Vitality - (B 23 and B 47)
Caution: Do not press on disintegrating discs or fractured bones.
Location: In the lower back, between the second and third lumbar vertebrae, 2 to
4 finger widths away from the spine at waist level.
Benefits: Strengthens immune system, relieves lower back aches and fatigue.

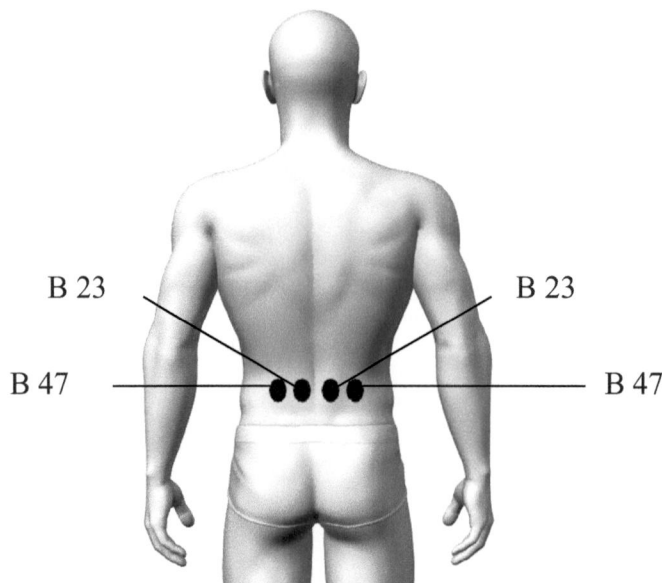

B 23   B 23

B 47   B 47

Sound Frequency Healing

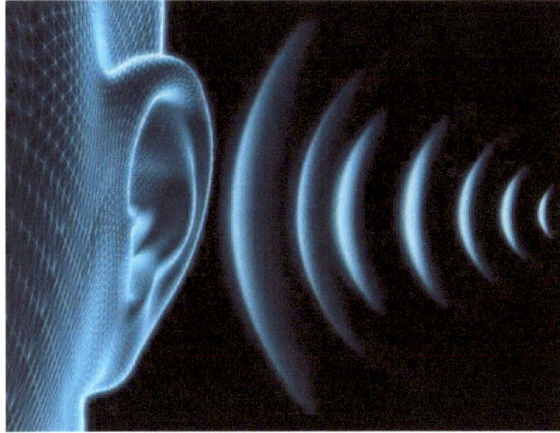

"Music is the movement of sound to reach the soul for the education of its virtue."
PLATO

Do you ever hear a piece of music or a sound in nature that seems to transport you to a place of bliss? How about a song that makes you feel playful? And what about the sound of car tires screeching or a dog barking all night? Those last examples can be very irritating or bring up feelings of dread and fear. The reason is, just as there are light wave frequencies, there are also multiple sound wave frequencies. Sound has a direct impact on our moods and brain-to-body response. They can have a calming, energetic or irritating effect on us.

A sound wave travels into a medium (in this case, the client's body as well as our own during the healing), by vibrating objects such as those listed on the following pages.

As the sound wave moves through our body, each particle of our body vibrates at the same frequency. There are also pitches in a sound wave, higher and lower, occurring as lighter or denser, shorter or longer waves and frequencies.

All frequencies and pitches are a part of our body's construction and just as our bodies contain lighter to denser auric compositions, specific pitches will resonate with specific areas of our body. Therefore, sounds that are harmonious (consonance) will relax our state of being, whereas dis-harmony (dissonance) will irritate us. Simplistically, these are agreeable or dis-agreeable effects.

Why Sound Heals

Sound waves travel through the body. Whenever there is an injury such as a pulled tendon, the outer muscles will tighten up in response to compensate and protect the injured area. Massage loosens up the outer muscles but sound waves loosen the internal muscles and connective tissues so blood flow can more easily feed the origin of the injury. Even ongoing stress can cause the constriction of tissues and blood flow thus creating aches, pain, and injury.

Throughout history, sounds have been an intricate thread used in spiritual and healing rituals. Hymns, chanting and drumming (music comprised of a harmonious vibration or cadence) elicited a harmonious effect on the congregation or individual. This not only relaxed tension in the body but also created an environment more conducive for a receptive, meditative state.

Once again, our ancient ancestors learned by observation that which we can now scientifically explain and measure.

How to use sound

In any healing, you can incorporate sounds. Again, only with practice and experimentation will you learn when and how to utilize these tools. All the various tools in the healer's tool box need to be introduced into the healing smoothly and appropriately. A healing must not be sporadic or jarring but rather a smoothing symphony from beginning to end.

Sound Tools: Good Vibrations

- **Rattle**: This is a Shamanic tool which can be used for waking up energies with an active stimulating effect. The *dis*sonant vibration will stir up *dis*harmony (the consciousness of *dis*ease) whereby physical, mental and emotional issues or awareness can then surface. I only use dissonant sounds at the beginning of a healing.

- **Tibetan Bowls:** Tibetan bowls will wake up the body's cellular consciousness but in a more agreeable way. I use these after the rattle.

- **Quartz Crystal Singing Bowl:** These bowls have a sound wave pressure that penetrates deeply into the tissues. These sound waves have a massaging result for the outer and inner muscles. The larger the bowl, the deeper/lower the pitch. Extremely effective in releasing the body armor.

One advantage of a large bowl is that you can add water to it to generate higher pitches. Different parts of the body resonate to different pitches and tones (lower half of the body responds to lower tones and the upper half to the higher). Lower to higher tones also correlate to the Chakra Totem.

- **Chimes:** Use soft, lighter pitch chimes near the end of a healing. The tones resonate to the upper chakras eliciting a peaceful meditative state.

- **Tuning Forks:** My favorite! If you can acquire a group of tuning forks with a range of pitches, do it. A complete range will cover all needs of the body. Every client I have used these on has said that they feel like they had just had a full body massage. I believe they are the epitome of effective sound therapy. Tuning forks carry the sound of the perfect 5th in pitch, an exponential vibration of harmony. I suggest that you contact us for instructions in using them properly.

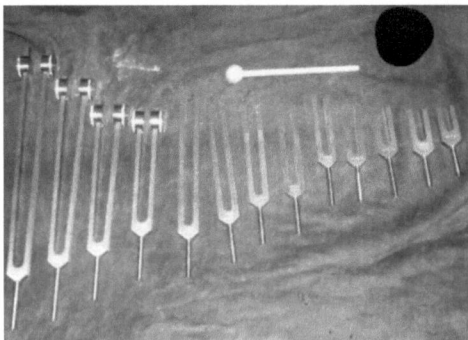

Tuning forks in graduating sizes

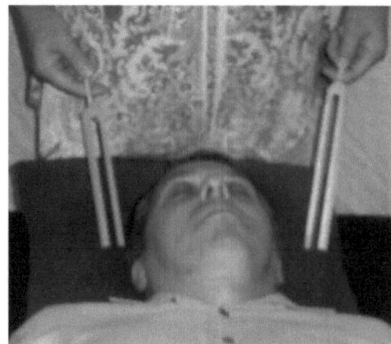

Using tuning forks with a client

- **Chanting:** Again, from ancient times, drumming, gourd rattling and singing have been used in healing. From lullabies to celebrations, prayer rituals to death ceremonies, the effects of sound have become an integral part of our spiritual expression. The utility of sounds ranges from general usage to a specific, designated purpose. The chanting of specific words or syllables creates harmony with meaning.

Most people are familiar with the image of the yogi, sitting in meditation and chanting "Om". It is believed that this sound is the sound of the universe and, by repeating it, the meditator merges with the frequency of the origins of existence, resulting in a harmonious state of oneness with all of creation above and below. Chanting is considered the seed, root and heights for spiritual development.

Chant #1

"*Om Mani Padme Hum*" (Sanskrit) is a mantra especially revered by the Dalai Lama devotees. Tibetan Buddhists believe that saying the mantra (prayer) out loud or silently to oneself invokes the powerful benevolent attention and blessings of Chenrezig, the embodiment of compassion. Viewing the written form of the mantra is said to have the same effect. Each of the six syllables corresponds with a meaning, chakra, color and human attribute (i.e. generosity, ethics, patience, diligence, wisdom) as well as human growth issues, (i.e. pride, envy, hatred). The mantra's purpose is to assist the chanter in transcending the negative consciousness to the higher consciousness of wisdom and peace.

Dilgo Khyentse Rinpoche's definition: *"The mantra Om Mani Padme Hum is easy to say, yet quite powerful, because it contains the essence of the entire teaching. When you say the first syllable Om, it is blessed to help you achieve perfection in the practice of generosity. The second syllable, Ma, helps perfect the practice of pure ethics, while the third, Ni, helps achieve perfection in the practice of tolerance and patience. Pa, the fourth syllable, helps to achieve perfection of perseverance. The fifth, Me, helps achieve perfection in the practice of concentration and the final, sixth syllable, Hum, helps achieve perfection in the practice of wisdom.*

"So, in this way, recitation of the mantra helps achieve perfection in the six practices from generosity to wisdom. The path of these six perfections is the path walked by all the Buddhas of the three times. What could then be more meaningful than to say the mantra and accomplish the six perfections?" [1]

Mantras are a fascinating study and I encourage anyone interested to research the practice and translations of syllables. I also suggest just trying it for 30 days, all day long. It is an easy commitment and a very interesting experience. I can almost guarantee you will feel a shift in your emotional and mental states which in turn aids in physical well being.

Chant #2

"*Lam Vam Ram Yam Ham Om NG*" These seven syllables correspond to the seven primary chakras, Lam being the vibration of the 1st (Root) chakra and each subsequent syllable matching each chakra rising from the root.

Place your hand on each chakra as you sing the syllable. Research the meaning of the mantra and concentrate on its purpose. This is an exercise of introduction. Once you become familiar with the meaning as a whole, simply sing it throughout the day, freely and frequently.

The use of these sound frequency healing tools is merely suggested. As with everything presented in this manual, take what you like and leave the rest.

---

[1] Dilgo Khyentse Rinpoche, *Heart Treasure of the Enlightened Ones*
http://en.wikipedia.org/wiki/Om_mani_padme_hum

Chant #3

As you grow spiritually you will develop your intuition. Since, like snowflakes- no two of us being the same- your unique connection with your spirit will also develop.

In Shaman Teachings, it is suggested that you find your own song and dance of personal expression and empowerment. You can ask in meditation to receive your own chant for your needs.

This takes no special skill or natural talent. The only things you need to find your chant are an open mind and patience. Through practice, it will come and it will reflect your true inner self, your spirit, as opposed to how you and others perceive you in the outside world.

I received a chant in a meditation. I did not ask for it. I was in turmoil at that time in my life. In my silent meditation with the intention of nothing more than "give me what I need for now", I heard a song in my mind. After the meditation, I recorded it on a tape recorder immediately. This was the chant/song:

Ah Ne Ma Ni
(Ah Nee Ma Nye)

Ah Ne Ma Ni

Ma Ne Ma Ni

Months later, I met a Hopi Native and I sang my chant song to him and asked him about it. He was surprised and said "It's like a lullaby. Ma Ne Ma Ni means *the mind of the outside and the mind of the inside, meet and bring you peace*." This was a gift to me as a confirmation of our ability to receive what we need through meditation. I use my personal chant often.

Record chants that may come to you in meditation. You can intuitively sense there meaning for you at this point in your life. *You* are your best interpreter.

_____

_____

_____

_____

_____

_____

_____

_____

_____

_____

_____

_____

Chant Meditation: Introduction

The sound vibration of each syllable will resonate through your body consciousness and meridians.

1. In a sitting meditation, keep your back straight (chakras aligned) and imagine each syllable you chant correlating with each chakra until the chant, body, mind and spirit merge into one flowing vibration. This will occur when mental and physical focus become effortless. At this point, enjoy the song-like quality of your chanting as your body, mind and spirit are now uniting on the same frequency.

2. After you've finished chanting, sit in silent meditation. This is the best part of sound frequency. After chanting you will feel the harmonious energies you have generated throughout your aura. This is the state of being where the healing takes place. Don't cheat yourself of optimum results. Continue to sit in the silence to allow wisdom and knowledge to come to you.

Chant for approximately 3-5 minutes. Then meditate for no less than 20 minutes.

Record your experiences after practicing each exercise on the following pages.

_____

_____

_____

_____

_____

_____

_____

_____

_____

_____

_____

_____

_____

_____

_____

_____

_____

_____

Chant Exercise: "Om Mani Padme Hum"

Position Exercise

1. Sit on a chair in an upright position.

2. Focus on each syllable associated with each chakra. Start at the Root Chakra (OM) and continue up the chakra totem.

3. Either rest your hands on your lap or join the tip of each thumb to the tip of your first fingers and rest your wrists on your knees. This yoga mudra closes the energy circuit, directing and transferring energy inward like a figure eight thereby promoting a deeper meditative experience.

OM circulates around the body

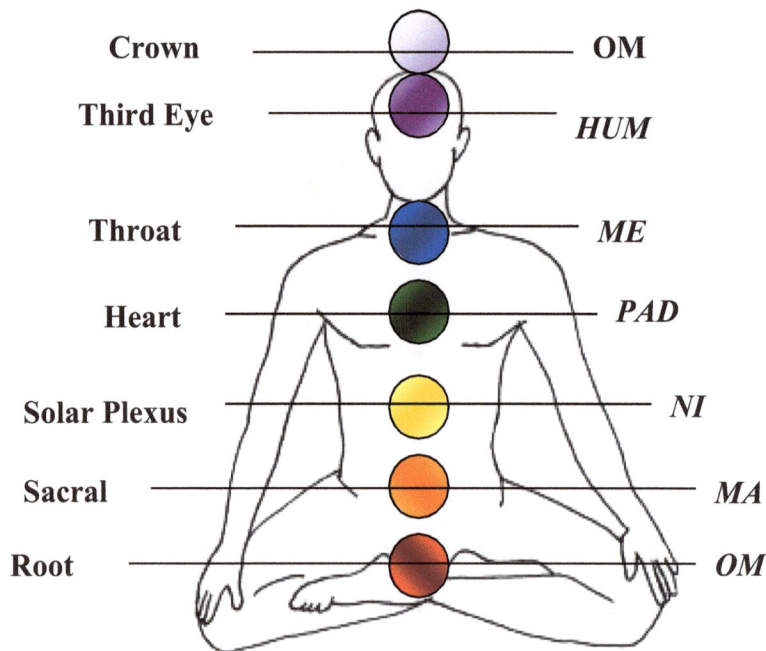

Crown	OM
Third Eye	HUM
Throat	ME
Heart	PAD
Solar Plexus	NI
Sacral	MA
Root	OM

Chant Exercise "Lam, Vam, Ram, Yam, Ham, Om, Ng"

Position Exercise

1. Sit on a chair or in an upright position.

2. Focus on and sing each syllable with each chakra. Start at the Root Chakra (LAM) and continue up the Chakra totem.

3. Either rest your hands on your lap or join the tip of each thumb to the tip of your first fingers and rest your wrists on your knees. This yoga mudra closes the energy current.

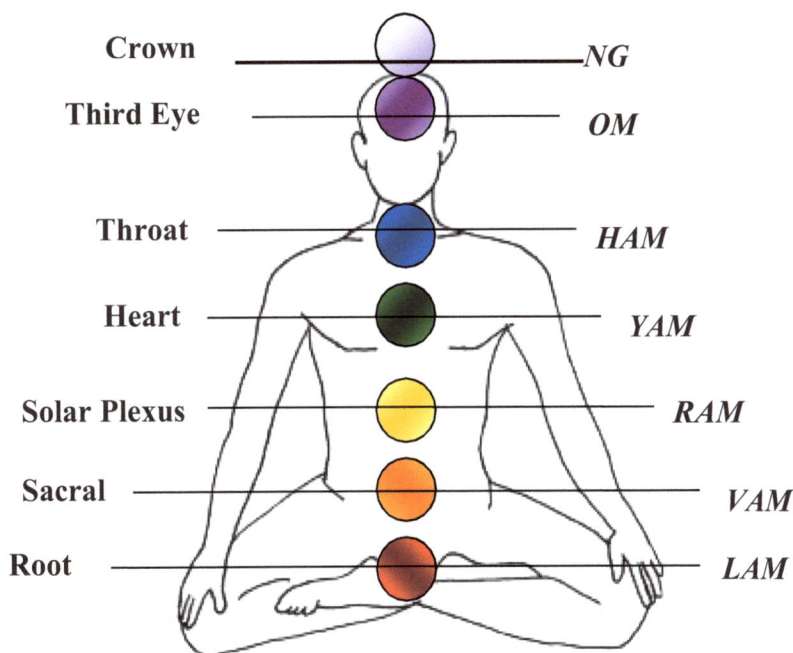

Chakra	Syllable
Crown	NG
Third Eye	OM
Throat	HAM
Heart	YAM
Solar Plexus	RAM
Sacral	VAM
Root	LAM

Chapter 9

Conversing with Consciousness

"Standing on the bare ground…
All mean egotism vanishes.
I become the transparent eyeball; I am nothing. I see it all;
The currents of the universal being circulated through me;
I am part and parcel with God."

RALPH WALDO EMERSON

Emotions and the Body

"Emotion always has it's roots in the unconscious and manifests itself in the body."
IRENE CLAREMONT de CASTILLIJO

Every body part is associated with our characteristics, attitudes and emotions. When we are negatively impacted for a length of time, the emotions will exhibit themselves as aches, pains and, eventually, dis-eases in the physical body. If we were to section the body off into quadrants (i.e.: front, back, left, right)and add the correlating aspects of each, they would look like this:

The Body Front & Back

Back:	Front:
Masculine "I do"	*Feminine "I perceive"*
How we show strength	*How we face the world*
Associated with the subconscious and/or hidden thoughts, feelings	*Associated with conscious thoughts, feelings*
Steadfast, achieving	*Wisdom, spiritual*
Outer pride, optimism	*Inner pride, healthy caution*
Stress, pain due to overburden	*Stress, pain due to fear, helplessness and inaction*
Giving too much, lack of receiving, rigid thinking	*Receiving too much, lack of giving enough*
Externally expressed anger from fear projected outward or trust in self and others	*Internally expressed depression, anger from fear held in or inner peace and self worth*

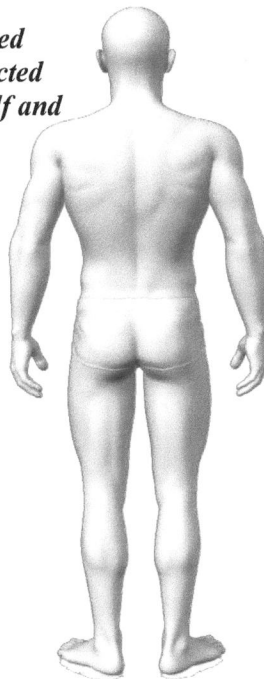

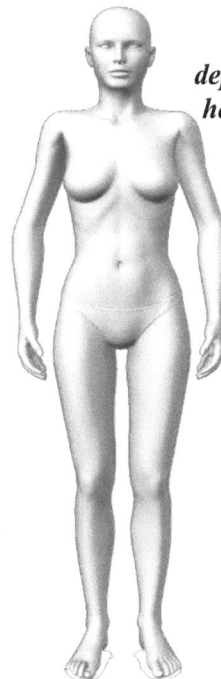

The Body Left & Right

Male

Right Side:

- *Masculine*
- *Giving*
- *Assertive/Aggressive*
- *Rational, Logical thinking*
- *Action oriented*
- *Stating*
- *Assessing*

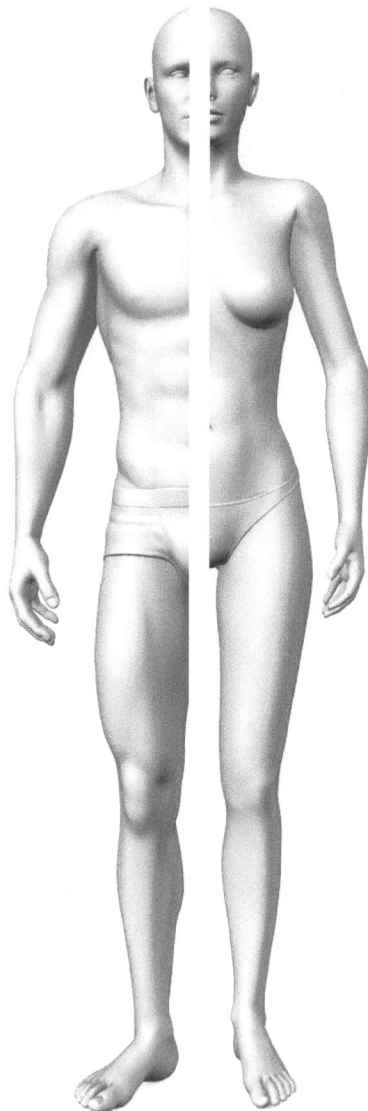

Female

Left Side:

- *Female*
- *Receiving*
- *Yielding, Passive*
- *Intuitive, Creative*
- *Growth oriented*
- *Reflecting*
- *Compassionate*

Utilizing and balancing both sides of our selves is the goal.

Head and Neck

Specific parts of the body (and the emotions or functions they relate to), when blocked or suppressed may manifest into physical imbalances. As an example, our ears. We may not want to hear what others have to say, even though the advice or concern is valid. So, we tune it out. Over the course of time we may develop an earache or hearing loss. Shown here are some of the emotional aspects related to individual body parts and chakra location.

Eyes: *How we view the world.*

Nearsighted = Introverted. Farsighted = extroverted. Wisdom, self-acceptance, clarity.

Nose: *Sense of smell connects to emotions, memories.*

Jaw: *Communication, determination, expression (speaking out).*

Neck: Throat Chakra, *where ideas and emotions merge. Self expression, speaking your truth, confidence.*

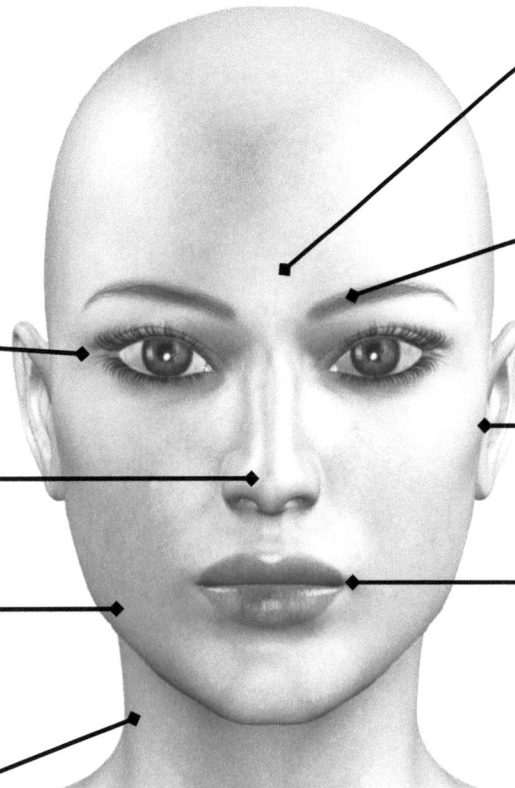

Forehead: Third Eye Chakra, *mental power, peace, worry, trust in intuition/faith.*

Brow: *expresses wonder, anger, concentration, confusion, intelligence, humor.*

Ears: *Willingness to hear the truth and other's opinions.*

Mouth: *How we take in sustenance (air, drink, food) and new information (food for thought, chew on this). Frown = low self-worth Tight-lipped = resistance.*

The Torso (Front)

Chest: Heart Chakra
love, relationship, breath, grief, depression, fear of living.

Stomach: Solar Plexus Chakra
emotional strength, confidence, coping, calm, addictions, control issues, anxiety. The 2nd power chakra.

Abdomen: Sacral Chakra
Trust, self-worth, empowerment, sexuality, guilt, shame. Our feminine side experiences digestive problems here. Our masculine side may experience back problems. The 1st power chakra.

Pelvis/Hips: Root Chakra
The "seat of the soul", survival, safety, reproductive organs, prostate, colon, uterus issues arise from fear of mortality.

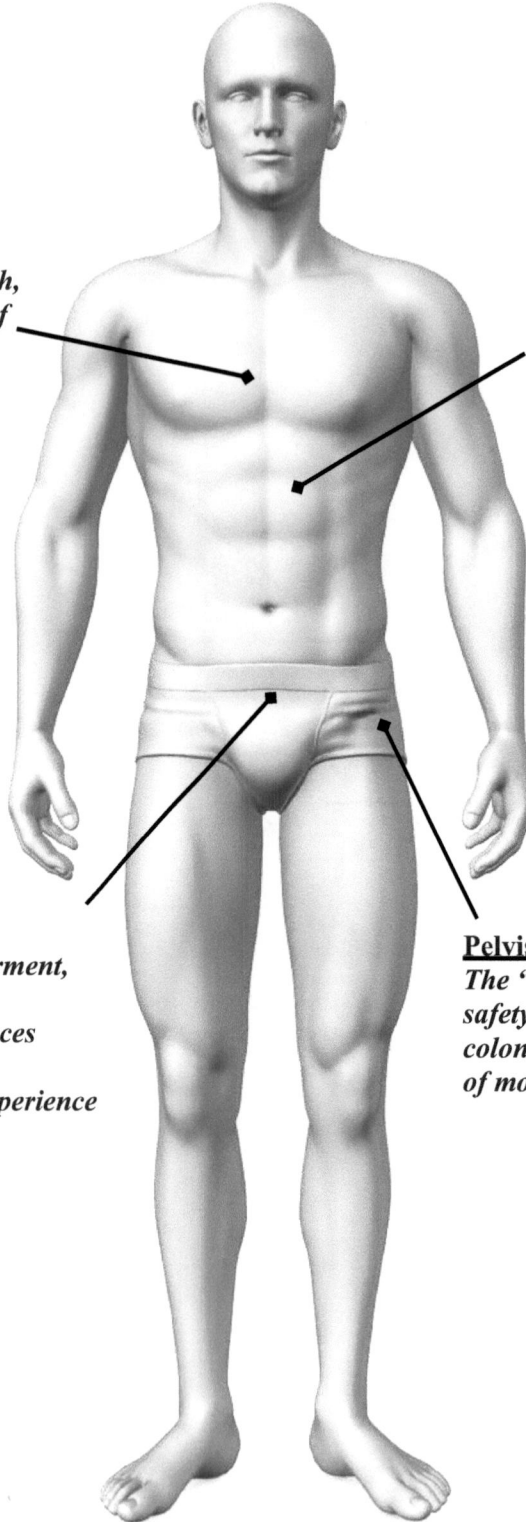

The Torso (Back)

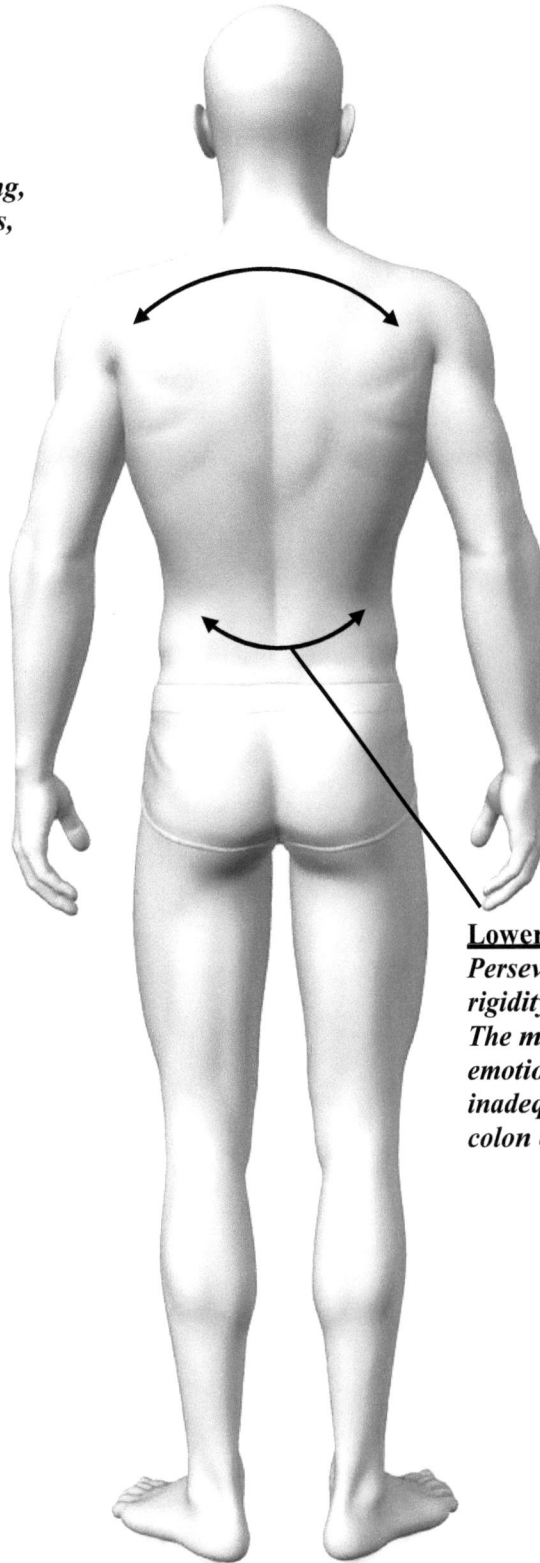

Upper Back:
Healthy pride, embracing, frustration, anger, stress, guarded, withdrawn.

Lower Back:
Perseverance, mental flexibility, rigidity.
The male side of us stores negative emotions, responsibility and inadequacy here. May manifest as colon or back problems.

The Extremities (Arms & Legs)

Shoulders:
Content, relieved, trusting others assistance, carrying the weight of the world, anxiety, migraines, neck/shoulder pain.

Arms & Hands:
Giving, receiving, protecting, expressing love from the Heart Chakra. The female of us holds control, anger and fear here.

Elbows:
Faith, flexibility, resistance. Holding too tightly to a person, relationship, or idea due to fear.

Feet:
Stability, standing your ground, being grounded, taking the next step, confusion/fear of committing to a path of action.

Knees:
Ability to move forward, letting go of rigid ego or old patterns, fear of change.

Ankles:
Turning points, decision making (which path to take in life), fear of decision making.

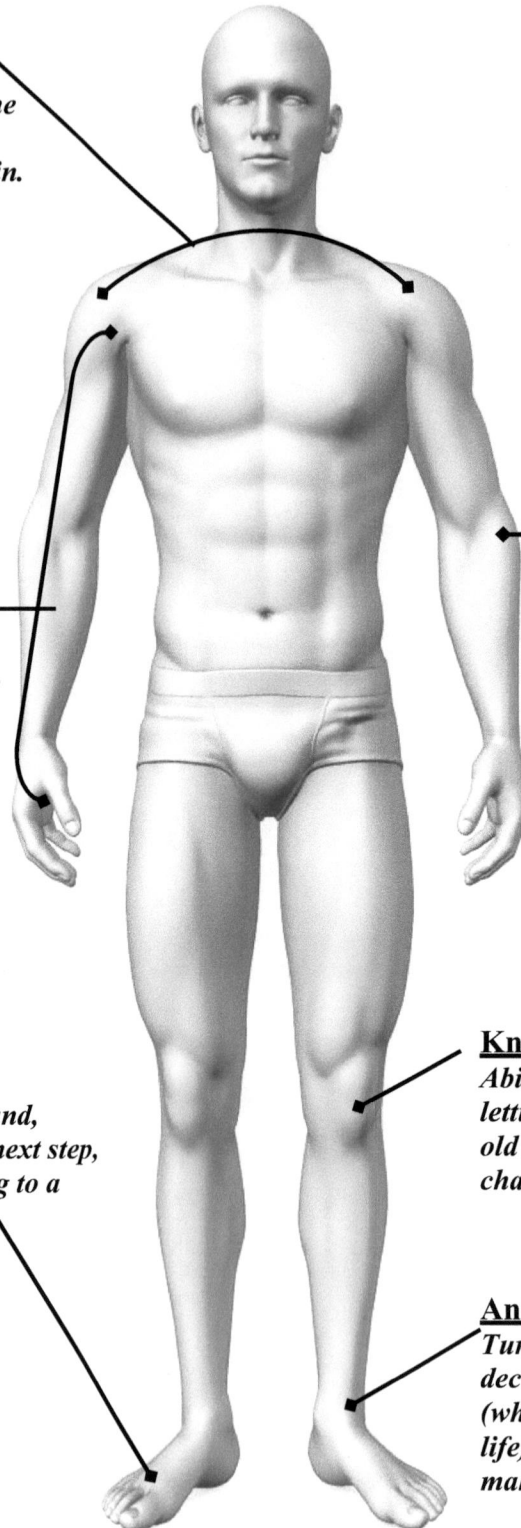

Internal Organs and Balancing

Organs, too, are a repository for emotions just like the other parts of the body. See the table below for the corresponding various emotions correlating to specific organs. Note that the organs are paired according to their complementary Yin/Yang nature.

Organs	Positive Emotions	Negative Emotions
Heart & Small Intestines	**Joy, fun, receptiveness**	**Shyness, over-seriousness**
Spleen & Stomach	**Sympathy, serenity**	**Resistance to change, apprehension**
Lungs & Large Intestines	**Clarity, communication, productivity**	**Fear, grief, indecision**
Kidneys & Bladder	**Calm, restful sleep, introspective, giving, energy**	**Fear, frustration, hoarding, over activity, lack of rest/sleep**
Liver & Gallbladder	**Enthusiasm, creativity, cleanliness in home and body**	**Anger, gluttony, being in a rut**

In a healing you can incorporate an **organ balancing** by laying each hand on each paired organ until you feel an equalization between the two, just as you do in the 20 Chakra Balancing.

You can do this on yourself as well, during your daily meditation.

Recommended Reading: <u>Staying Healthy with the Seasons</u> by Elson M. Haas, M.D.

This book is an excellent guide from Chinese Natural Medicine. It explains the associations of these five paired organs to the five seasons (Autumn, Winter, Spring, Summer and Late Summer), as well as the specific foods to eat during each.

I have found it to be a wealth of information and often give clients handouts from it according to the season their appointment is scheduled.

God is Here at Home in
Mind-Body

"God is a word, however problematical, we do not have to look up in the dictionary.
We seem to have its acquaintance from birth."
JOHN UPDIKE

We often look outside ourselves for the answers to the mysteries of life and death, particularly if consciousness exists after death. We too often seek ways to escape what seems like a mundane reality or attempt to experience a different and better reality.

Because being human can sometimes feel very lonely, we search for something that can bring us a sense of connectedness and significance to this reality which we call human and to this body which we call home. And, amidst the 360° backdrop of unending overwhelm called the Universe, we feel small. Hence, Man's search for God.

But when we seek connection outside of ourselves, we actually separate ourselves more. It is a human experience to feel separation from the greater God- consciousness. In fact, it is the very reason we have chosen to incarnate- to bring God to ourselves and our planet to help each other and enjoy our spectacular existence; to expand our consciousness and continue to create more just as our parent universe creates and expands. Yes, we are its microscopic clone. We are the universe and every answer we seek is right here at home within every atom of our being, literally.

It is so wonderful to see our society reawakening to our innate ability to reconnect to our source. Meditation, of course has been one avenue to do so and is essential as a foundation for other pathways as well. Yet I have found that in our society, there is also a valid need for more tools and more readily apparent results. There is nothing wrong with needing to get there sooner or needing confirmation or validation for the work of faith and science. The work that follows is part faith and part science. They work in tandem, complimenting each other as we walk along this human path.

Especially in our society, where technology is moving faster than our spiritual maturity and awareness, there is a need to learn and catch up quickly. Therefore, the more skilled we are in tapping into the answers to who we are, the more capable we become in making the right decisions in our daily and global life. We need to, because separation equals fear and anger; knowledge consequently equals confidence and peace. Keep in mind that living this life is a constant endeavor to balance the myriad of aspects that make that life.

Our society needs a sense of personal confidence on a soulful level. God is not someone who saves us at the last minute. God begins here at home, in our own existence. Your own living consciousness is God living and residing there.

So, how do you tap into that knowledge – cell knowledge- and the undeniable rewards of its comfort and security, knowing we are safe, complete and never alone again?

How do you pick up the phone and ask the God-consciousness the many questions of your life and purpose and how do you get a reply? *Start by talking to your cells.*

Consciousness exists in every cell. Energy itself, with all the experience carried with it, doesn't know the difference between the past, present or future. Energy simply exists. This is the basic truth of Quantum physics. Therefore, all information is available to us if we seek it within ourselves through meditation, including mind-body dialogue.

Mind-Body Dialogue

Ask

At first this exercise may be a challenge because it may feel a bit silly asking your body to respond to you as if it could talk. But it does. Every discomfort, every twinge or pain, is your body trying to communicate to you that something is out of balance within it. The more you practice this exercise, the more effectively you will communicate with your body. Pay close attention to the answers. There will be distinct answers, not a vague pain or twinge that you logically correlate as the result of some activity. This connection is more than merely physical. You are now consciously merging the physical body with the emotional and spiritual body.

Close your eyes and begin to meditate. Ask your body-being which part wants or needs to speak. Perhaps your liver stings in response. The mind-to-body dialogue may go something like this:

Question: *Ask your body to tell you how he or she feels.*
Answer: Your liver may, like an inner child, say, "I am angry and I need for you to stop talking to so and so", (a relationship that is not healthy anymore).
Question: *"What do you need me to do?"*
Answer: "I (liver) need you to tell the truth and then I need a long walk in the woods so I can breathe."

Another example: Issue - Your lungs respond with tightness.
Question: *"Tell me how you feel?"*
Answer: "Scared! I am overwhelmed at work!"
Question: *"What do you need me to do for you?"*
Answer: "Breathe more and slow down"

This dialogue can go on for quite a while if you are really present and not judging the experience. During this exercise and whenever you meditate for any reason (personal self-growth or healing), remember to leave the logical, thinking brain behind until you're done. The logical mind houses the ego. As we go through our daily routines (working, housekeeping, driving), we live with the ego in the forefront. Generally, we are so comfortable with it showing us what we *want* to see that we miss what is truly happening. To connect to the Divine is to bypass the ego, to gain a deeper, truer understanding of ourselves and the world around us. The "we know what's best" view of the world is not necessarily accurate. With the ego put aside, we may see the situation for what it truly is: a learning experience from and with the Divine for our spiritual and emotional growth.

You can continue to talk to all the parts of your body and ask profound questions. Each different area of the body carries a different package of information. Try it! Be imaginative, free and bold. Ask about the beginning of life if you want. Ask about a loved one on the other side. All information is available because you *are* the universe in a shell, that is all and that is everything.

Mind-body dialogue is truly fascinating. I have seen the practice transform people's fears and victim mentality into empowerment and purpose. I have seen them expose the meaning of their illness, which has led to the answers for recovery.

Life

The creative forces continually seek balance. This homeostasis results in good health. The ingredients to re-balance are here at "home" where life resides and its voice speaks from your life force body, from your energy system which carries consciousness and the imprints of the creative force. Whatever is required to balance the body, mind, emotions and spirit is available.

Cell

Consciousness may tell you to drink some orange juice right now; to soak up some negative ions at a waterfall; to work through an old abuse issue; exercise; pray or meditate. With daily practice, mind-body dialogue becomes synergistic. Focusing on consciousness creates more of it and is multifaceted in action and results. Eventually, you are not just practicing a technique, but *living* it, *being* it. Every moment of every day you are tuned in.

As you experience the life-changing process, the expanded consciousness emanates from your energy field to the energy fields of others you meet in life. Sometimes their energy fields will resonate with yours, resulting in changes for them. Their energies remember innate health and will seek balance to restore it. My favorite saying is: ***"As you heal, we all heal."***

Mind-body dialogue is just one way to bring consciousness home. Whatever avenue you choose, apply it. It is only the action of a philosophy that creates its' reality. Bring all you seek back home. Your truths are right here and the reality of your existence is very far from mundane.

Incorporating Mind-Body Dialogue as a Healer

Always ask your client ahead of time if they would like you to incorporate this technique in their healing. Some clients do not want to delve into the psyche or to feel uncomfortable emotions they're not ready to face. With time, they may become able to trust themselves and you enough to try.

Do not start out with this technique, but rather, integrate it about half-way into the healing. The remainder of the healing can then re-center and relax the client. Adding a few affirmations related to the mind-body dialogue discoveries, after the negative extraction, can be an empowering experience for them.

Three Basic Questions:

    1. *"What do you feel?"*
    2. *"What do you need from me?"*
    3. *"What can we agree on?"*

I usually begin the mind-body dialogue after the polarity balancing chakra section, steps 1-8, before the shoulder, hip, knee, ankle and closing section. After the hands-on healing of the chakras, I take my hands off the client and begin the mind-body dialogue. (It is important that you do not touch a client during a mind-body dialogue. Any outside stimuli will distract their inner journey and influence their answers.)

Here are some client sessions as examples:

Stacy

Me: "OK Stacy, first I want you to focus your concentration on your head, eyes, ears, neck and shoulders. Now, notice your right shoulder, elbow and wrist. Now, notice your left shoulder, elbow and wrist. Is there any discomfort in any area so far? Just say yes or no".

Stacy: "No."

Me: "Good. Now, take notice of your back, from top to bottom. Now, notice your right hip and knee and ankle. Now, notice your left hip, knee and ankle. Now Stacy, become aware of all the organs in your body: your throat, lungs, heart, liver, spleen, stomach, kidneys and intestines. Now Stacy, from head to toe, back to front and side to side, inside and out, what part of your body wants your attention?"

Stacy: "I don't know, I feel so relaxed right now."

Me: "That's great that you feel relaxed, Stacy. What part of your body bothers you when you're not this relaxed?"

Stacy: "My stomach"

Me: "OK. Now, ask your stomach to tell you everything she feels, like an inner child is telling you."

Stacy: Pauses, "Tight and upset."

Me: "Good. Ask the stomach what she specifically feels like ; angry, afraid, sad, hurt?" (I will suggest these choices of emotions only when I have to).

Stacy: "Angry!"

Me: "Great. Now ask the stomach to tell you why it's angry."

Stacy: Pauses, "It says it's always hungry and so angry."

Me: "Why is it always hungry?"

Stacy: "Because I don't eat much."

Me: "Why don't you eat much?"

Stacy: "I'm so upset all of the time."

Me: "OK, what is upsetting you now?"

Stacy: "My husband is so mean and scares me."

Me: "OK, Stacy, so go ask your stomach now if it's afraid?"

Stacy: "Yes! Always a nervous wreck."

Me: "All right, now ask the stomach what it needs from you as it's parent, guardian."

Stacy: Long pause "Help, it just wants out. To get away from him, but I can't."

Me: "Good. Now let's understand, there's a conflict between wanting out and not being able to get out, is that right?"

Stacy: "Yes."

Me: "So you can't tell your stomach 'OK, I'll get you out right now,' is that correct?"

Stacy: "Yes."

Me: "So okay, what one step can you agree on to start easing and nurturing the stomach's needs? Support groups, therapy, taking a class, a hobby, someone you can talk to… just one simple step. Ask your stomach now".

Stacy: Pause, "It says it wants me to go to therapy."

Me: "Ok, now, will you do that?"

Stacy: "Yes."

Me: "Does your stomach believe you?"

Stacy: Pause, "No."

Me: "Good, then what's the next possibility to agree on, just as a first step? Talk to your stomach, Stacy."

Stacy: Pause, "The minister, the minister at my church, I will talk to him."

Me: "Does your stomach believe you?"

Stacy: "Yeah."

She breathes out a big sigh of relief at the time. This is often the signal that the inner and outer conflict is released, when the authentic self is unified.

Once this was accomplished, I told Stacy to take a few breaths and relax while I continued the healing session.

When a mind-body dialogue is this intense, I will guide the client into one of the relaxing imageries and re-establish a peaceful healing state, allowing her body and mind to rest. I will light incense again and take all the time needed for the client to feel spiritually nourished. I may suggest an affirmation while I'm closing the session, such as "I am guided, I am safe, I am not alone."

Please practice this technique on yourself and friends or family before you work with clients. Practice is essential. If a client exhibits serious distress then gently stop the process saying, "This is good information, Stacy. You can let it go now and we will talk later. Now, just enjoy the comfort of the healing."

Some mind-body dialogues are quick and clear, as in the following example.

Kevin

Kevin was worried because his whole body ached. His muscles were weak and he was always tired. When he asked his muscles how they felt, they said, "Mad and tired as hell". When he asked them what they needed him to do, the response was "Please give me water and orange juice!"

After the healing, I asked Kevin how much water or juice he usually drank and he answered, "I can't even tell you". It was actually *zero* and we laughed.

Kevin replaced his four sodas a day with a mixture of water and orange juice. He'd fill several bottles for work each day. Now, he calls it his "Elixir of Life".

Past Life Mind-Body Dialogue

There are instances when a client has been diligent with their health regimen and still can't seem to get better. Many times, this is the natural cycle of life and aging.

Sometimes however, if it is in a client's belief system, a chronic condition is an echo of a past life occurrence.

Barry

"I have had a pain the middle of my back for as long as I can remember." This was Barry's complaint at our first meeting.

After several healings without improvement, I suggested he ask his back if this pain was connected to other life times.

Immediately, Barry let out a grunt and one of his legs kicked. He laughed and said "Well, I guess so."

We proceeded with a past-life regression. In a nutshell, Barry had been stabbed to death (in the back) by the husband of a woman he had been having an affair with sometime in the 18th century.

Barry had continued this behavior in his present life. He was so disturbed and awakened by this experience that he sought counseling. As a result, he stopped cheating and after a few months the back pain went away.

All we've experienced from our past lives, all we experience today and all that we will experience in the future, has been, is and will be recorded in cellular memory.

In all the years of implementing body-mind dialogue in healing sessions, very rarely have I witnessed a client who did not experience a positive outcome from it.

I still find it fascinating and I practice it almost daily in my own life.

Cellular Memory Imagery

After using the mind-body dialogue, you have assisted a client with an acute or chronic condition in identifying the body part along with the issue. They have come to understand the issue intellectually and emotionally. The client has followed through with the agreements made with the inner and outer self. The next step is Cellular Memory Exercise. This will further the clients healing and allow them to work on their dis-ease between healing sessions.

The Healthy Cell Imagery

1. Relax and breathe deeply as you count down from 20 to 1, slowly and patiently.

2. Now, ask your consciousness to see a *healthy cell*, as if with a camera lens. Don't force it. Let it happen. It is innate knowledge.

3. Once you see it as if through a camera lens, *zoom in* as close as you can and observe the healthy cell. See its movement, light, texture, energy, vitality and beauty.

4. Now, hold it lovingly in your hands and feel its life-force. It is spectacular. This is how stunning you are.

5. Relax with this image for as long as you want. Watch what happens. You are just observing.

The Unhealthy Cell Imagery

1. Next, ask your consciousness to see an *unhealthy* cell. Just allow the image to come to you.

2. Now, zoom in as close to it as you can and observe its details in movement, texture and energy.

3. Next, hold it lovingly in your hands and feel its emotions; it's state of being.

4. Ask this unhealthy cell *where exactly* it resides in your body. There may be many, however the most important will be the first area that comes to mind.

5. Proceed with the mind-body dialogue. After you've come to an agreement, say this to that body part daily during your meditations:

Tell the unhealthy cells "Thank you for the warning. You can heal now". Replace them with beautiful healthy cells. Imagine this happening, one at a time, zooming in until the entire area of the body part is filled with vibrant healthy cells. Then, imagine these healthy cells spreading throughout your entire body and aura.
State without a doubt: *"You are healed and healthy now, so be it."*

A Tid-Bit on Past Lives
The many layers of existence

"People like us, who believe in physics, know that the distinction between past, present and future is only a stubbornly persistent illusion."

ALBERT EINSTEIN

In reality, there are no past, present or future lives. They are all happening at the same time. We can only perceive time in a linear fashion. But time is anything but linear.

In our present-time experience (at least theoretically) physicists and mathematicians state that mathematically there are 11 dimensions of existence, just four of which are perceived by human beings. Only three of those are physically experienced by people: height, width and depth. The fourth dimension is time.

According to Einstein, space/time is not in motion but, rather, *we* are in motion through it. Therefore, all moments of time (past, present and future) co-exist *simultaneously*.

Previous, current and impending lives are all part of one entity's or person's chain of reality which produces a myriad of chains of reality.

No two entities can pursue the same chain of reality and thus cannot experience the same life, past, present or future. However, separate chains of reality can co-exist in parallel during the same period as we understand it (i.e. 19th century, 15th century etc.)

Essentially, this means that two or more separate entities or people can experience past, present or future lives together.

In terms of past-life memory, the experience which had the most impact on a person's greater consciousness (the collective multidimensional experience) can be resonating with a person's "present" conscious life.

Consequently, in past-life regressions, any issue carried over, needing resolve or order will surface. Therefore our present choices are so important.

Every choice we make in the here-and-now effects our whole existence, our souls' evolution, our multi-dimensional course. Whether that be chaos or order will be determined by the choice. Not only are we interconnected to and thus affecting all those around us, we are also affecting all the facets of our multi-dimensional selves.

By revealing past-life issues in our present life, we are changing our future in this present life, as well as reuniting our souls' split consciousness. Unity above and below, so to speak, is the goal of every soul and ultimately in reuniting with God.

Negative Extractions: Introduction

What do you do with all those negative vibes you've accumulated over the years, maybe still lingering from childhood, from relationships, past lives or painful experiences overall?

Our auric fields are intermingling with others' constantly. Energy cords eventually grow and intertwine between us and those we spend a lot of time with. These connections may be positive and/or negative. Although an exceedingly negative person may finally be out of our lives, a residual energy cord attachment can remain, sometimes for years.

This can give the sensation of an undercurrent of depression or a physical weight even though we are progressing and enjoying much of our life.

With prolonged exposure, negativity will *energetically* get stuck on us. This consciousness builds upon itself, creating attached thought forms that we carry without realizing it. For example: As a child, you may have been called pudgy, big boned, or even fat. As an adult, you may be completely physically fit, however, those comments, those *thought forms,* have attached to you and you've carried them into your adult life. So instead of believing that you are fit and healthy, you still think of yourself as "a little overweight".

Since energy follows thought, these residual thought forms just need to be told where to go. A healer's deliberate intention can release them. Hundreds of my clients have said the same things after a Negative Extraction: "Wow, I feel so much lighter" and "Wow, everything looks brighter". I still find it extraordinary, every time I hear it.

The following "Negative Extraction Technique" may seem pretty farfetched but if this book so far has made sense to you, then this will too and in fact, you will see how it connects to the final dot, like the finale in a symphony. That is why it is the last technique presented in this manual. It is also the most difficult technique to perform effectively.

This procedure must be done without effort or ego, along with perfect timing and verbal cuing. This process of literal "energy exchange" is an art to perform.

You will know if you administered it correctly or not by your client's feedback. If they didn't say something on the order of "Holy Moly, that was incredible. I felt like I was out of my body", then keep practicing.

Because this technique is so tricky I offer training sessions by appointment. My contact information is in the back of this manual.

It can be difficult to perform this without having experienced it for yourself first. So, again, practice with a friend, both giving and receiving this transcendental healing.

Negative Extraction Technique: Step by Step Photos

After a complete healing and *before* the final closing segment is the right time for a Negative Extraction.

After the healing you will be well aware of what chakra your client's having difficulty with. That chakra will be the "weed spot" ready for extraction. Whenever in doubt, focus either on the Solar Plexus (which is the most common area) or on the Throat and Heart chakras. These chakras hold on to negative energy cords most often. We'll use the Solar Plexus as our example.

Negative Extraction on the Solar Plexus

1. After the healing:
Place your right hand on their Solar Plexus. Make a fist, as if you are grabbing hold of the stems of a weed. Let your client feel the weight of your fist and *do not* take it off the body as you continue on to the next step.

2. With your left hand, use your fingertips, as if you are gathering threads, starting from the toes, then up the leg, over the hips and into your fist on the Solar Plexus. Let your client feel you doing this. Gather up one leg, then the other. Repeat the process on the arms, starting with the fingertips, then up the arm to the shoulder. Gather up one arm and then the other, both to the fist. Then gather around the head and chest to the fist.

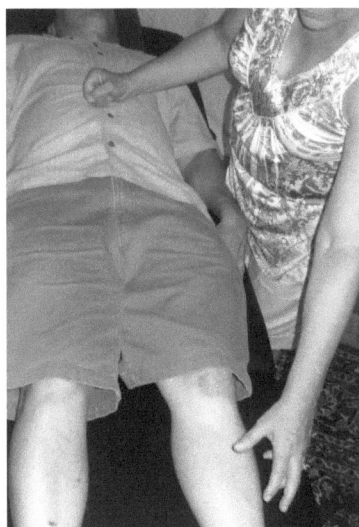

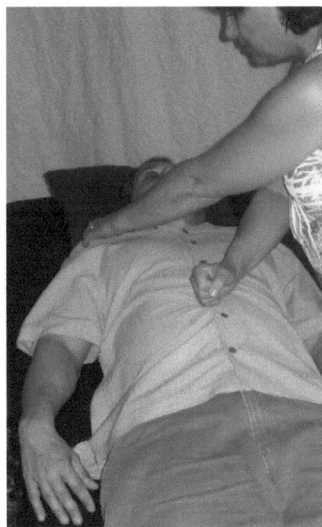

Gathering the "Threads"

Do this a few times while you verbalize the following:

A. Healer: *"Ok (client's name), I'm going to gather up all the negative energies that do not belong to you anymore. This may be stuff from other people from the past or present or old issues that you may have already worked on. All the energies that no longer serve you all gathering to this spot."*

B. Keep sweeping along the body, gathering to your fist and continue.

> **Healer:** *"Now (client's name), when you're ready, please nod and then I'm going to pull these attachments off, on the count of 3 ok?"*

237

Be quiet and patient then slowly stop gathering when your client nods the ok.
Press your fist firmly into the Solar Plexus and count out loud

Healer: *"1, 2, 3"*. On "3", you will do two things simultaneously. *1. Quickly release* your fist as if you are pulling out the roots of a hearty weed. Pull off all the cords 3 times swiftly and quietly fling them out and away from your client.

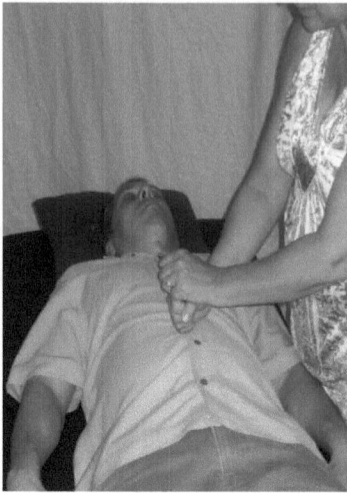

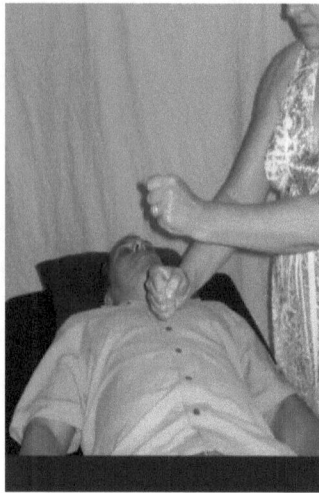

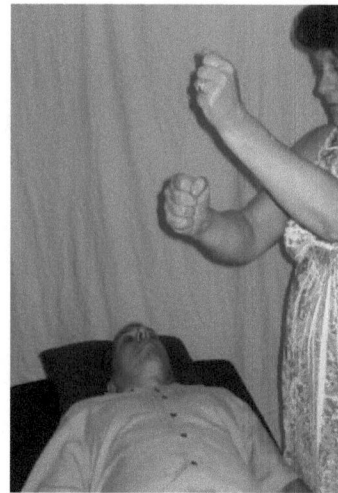

"Threads" gathered at the center being pulled off.

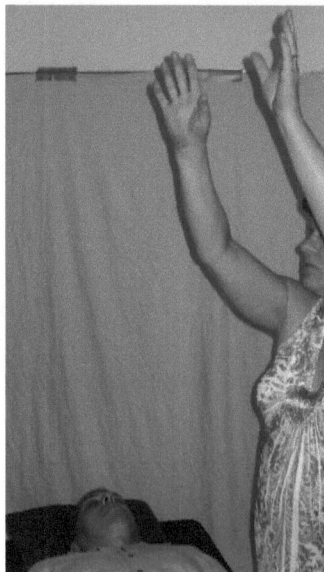

Releasing the "Threads".

2. At the same time, while you're doing this say:

Healer: *"I give this to Great Spirit* (God, or the universe, depending on your client's beliefs) *never to return"*.
Repeat this each time you pull them off (3 times total- 3 pulls, along with the statement each time). Then ask your client to repeat this statement once:

Client: *"I give this to Great Spirit, never to return"*.
   This participation empowers them with that simple statement, *"never to return"*. They are setting a mental and energetic statement barring negative energies from reconnecting to them. They are taking the responsibility for their own healing and establishing healthy boundaries.

D. After your client repeats this, *immediately* place your left palm warmly and lightly on the Solar Plexus and your right palm **above** your client's Crown Chakra and say very quietly, serenely and **slowly**, almost in a hypnotic whisper:

Healer: *"Now, we always replace the old with the new. So, imagine a beautiful new waterfall of color and light filling your body, carrying your true soul's energy of freedom, health, joy and love. <u>Hear the words:</u> "I am whole. I am new. I am worthy".*

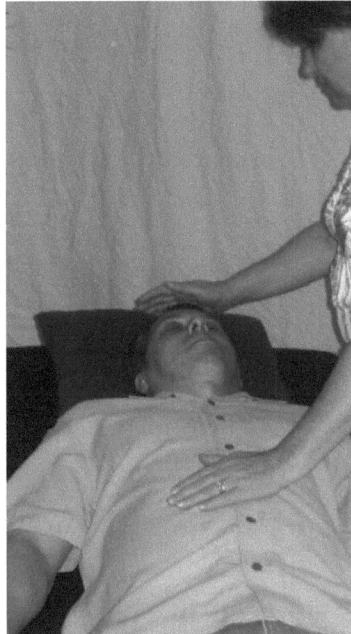

"Replacing the old with the new".

E. Lift your hands off gently and **say nothing more**. **Do nothing**. Do *not* disturb your client *in any way*. Quietly step away a few feet to allow an uninterrupted experience. (If you paced this procedure correctly, you will see the transformation on your client's face. You may observe a tranquil countenance, a younger appearance, or perhaps a glow and your client should be in a near-trance-like, peaceful state.)

F. Wait until the client comes back on his own. At that point, quietly finish the session with the usual closing-up sequence.

More is definitely not better

If your client didn't experience a definite shift of some kind, you may have talked too much, too loudly or too quickly. Remember, the words spoken to the client during the extraction need to be nearly whispered to maintain their deep theta hypnotic state.

Stick to this script. It works. I have had students who added affirmations during the energy exchange (the waterfall segment) and, by doing so, it snapped the client back to the present and lost the out-of-body kind of experience it should be.

After the extraction, the body is energetically open, the consciousness is expanded beyond the physical and the new energy (waterfall) is the soul (higher consciousness) merging and entering the body. This is *literally* an energy exchange, the negative being removed and the positive replacing it.

Notice that nowhere in the script am I extracting anything *specific*. There are no suggestions of taking away a specific person's negative energy or an explicit event or memory. There is a significant reason for this. The statement *"all negative energies that do not belong to you"*, as written, carries no particular expectations.

239

More so, any negative energies that *do* belong to the client are his issues still to be worked on and learned from to grow and will remain after the extraction. We do not *lose* by having negative attachments. We *learn*. Again, please stick to the script.

This is the "cherry on top" of a healing, a powerful transformational, blissful experience. For the recipient, it can truly feel like you've met your soul and your true self.

A final note

I only apply this technique when I feel a strong spiritual guidance to do so. I may only do this once or twice a year for a regular client. Think about that.

You will have many tools in your toolbox and you will be tempted to "play" with them to impress others or perhaps have the desire to share a cool tool. It's normal and we all go through it.

There will be plenty of times where you will have to learn when to back off and trust only what spirit directs.

As I continue to develop my skills and art as a healer and allow myself to be led by what I know and don't know, I find repeatedly now that the phrase "less is more" is the Truth. Even today, I am still learning to let go and let God.

Healing Stories

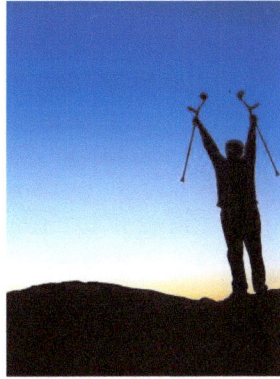

As a healer, you will undoubtedly encounter many types of clients with a myriad of ailments. Here are a few stories of my experiences with clients.

Peggy: A former client of mine named Peggy has muscular dystrophy, with episodes of stiffening muscle areas occurring about four to five times a year. When she came to me, she had already been involved in holistic therapies. She ate a healthy diet, exercised and used homeopathy. She had an optimistic attitude and a zest for learning. After a year of healing sessions, meditations, imagery and hypnotherapy direction, her episodes decreased to one a year. This was 18 years ago and she's still doing well.

John: Another client of mine, John, was a mountain climber. On one outing, a boulder fell on him, breaking his collar bone, an arm, some ribs and he lost his spleen, as well. In five sessions, I taught him pain and stress relief imagery techniques along with healings and aromatherapy work. A few months later, when I bumped into him, he said he uses the techniques and oils all the time and it has made a difference in pain reduction and recovery.

Tina: Tina was 21 years old with Crohn's disease, a very painful and debilitating intestinal condition. She inherited the gene from her family lineage. At the time I met her, she had not been able to work or continue her college studies for an entire year. She had lost a dangerous amount of weight and had approximately 20 diarrhea episodes a day. She was diligent with her diet but refused to take medication. I saw her once a week for healing and specific imageries and, within six weeks, she was back in school and her episodes decreased to four a day. She did her imagery every day and night and that is what it takes. She was determined to take responsibility for her own healing.

Diane: Diane was 53 years old. She had been an incest survivor and had undergone many years of therapy which had helped her greatly. She was functioning well yet living a daily life of fear. Initially, I refrained from leading her into an inner-child imagery, fearing a traumatic re-occurrence. But silent meditations were disturbing for her and the stress reduction techniques were simply not enough. I decided to offer and explain to her the inner child imagery. She said, "Let's do it." As I guided her in the imagery process to meet and converse with her inner wounded child, she could pinpoint the age of her psychic trauma. I then guided her to bring back the child she was at that age with her to a safe place. She said she saw an angel who took the child to the loving grandparent's home she remembered visiting periodically. She saw herself as that child, safe and happy. Whenever Jackie got afraid, she used this imagery and it worked for her. She said that all the years in therapy had helped her, but this imagery experience had been the only thing that diminished the undercurrent of terror she was feeling. Jackie will always have to cope with the emotional damage caused by the incest she experienced but, for her, the imagery process removed at least one negative emotional force from her life.

I have taught hundreds of people a variety of imagery techniques, dealing with issues including childhood traumas, addiction, injuries, emotional problems, post-traumatic stress, depression, anxiety, fear and hopelessness; physical issues, such as those that result from chemotherapy and radiation therapy and diseases like fibromyalgia and muscular dystrophy. I have seen the power of our beautiful minds at work first hand.

The additional benefit of practicing meditation and imagery is the development of patience. Once you have experienced peace of mind, inner calm and relief of stress, you want to maintain it. Ignorance is not bliss when you're suffering. Learning is exciting and motivating because your life changes in ways you never thought possible.

Patrick: Patrick has rheumatoid arthritis. He has had bi-weekly sessions with me for several years now. We start with a few simple yoga stretches and end with Qi Gong, an exercise of Chinese origin. In my healing work with Patrick, I have incorporated every tool in this manual over the years, according to his needs in any given session.

After a few years, I asked Patrick, "With such a chronic disease, how have these sessions helped you?" His answer was, "I can tell this helps, because when I've skipped a few weeks, I hurt more."

It always touches my heart when I hear these words from clients. It has so often kept me going when I doubted, at times, the validity of this unconventional work. At present, after over 2 decades of this work, I no longer doubt. I have seen so many people benefit, not just physically, but also in their personal expansion of awareness, of their body-mind connection. They become more in tune with themselves on an ever-increasing, regular basis.

Lisa: Lisa is 64 years old. She had an infection after a hysterectomy. The infection was resistant to antibiotics. She had an open hole in her abdomen the size of a baseball. Six weeks had gone by and she was lethargic, unable to work and said she felt like she was dying. Lisa had been a highly energetic and successful woman, but at this point, she could barely get up to feed herself. She had been in and out of the hospital because of fever and pain, yet the infection was growing. Her co-worker referred her to me. (This was one of the few house calls I've made, because she was too weak to drive.)

By the time I saw her, she was yellow from jaundice, despondent and she had lost a lot of weight. When I first saw her open, infected wound, I was frankly appalled she wasn't in the hospital right then and there. Lisa had no knowledge or interest in holistic therapies but allowed me to come by at the urging of her co-worker.

I gave here a crash course on what I would do and asked her if she was willing to try. I proceeded with Magnetic Polarity healing and Nature Imagery. Magnetic work pulls out infections and aides in regenerating healthy cell production.

The next day, she called to tell me what happened. After the healing, she said she slept like a baby. In the morning she had tons of energy and she couldn't believe it. Within 3 days, the infection flushed out of the wound and healing began. She was fine thereafter.

Yes, sometimes a healing like this occurs. In this case, the timing was significant. The infection she had was at the crucial point of metastasizing throughout her body which could have killed her. Because the infection was still localized and the body was so weak, the energy work was able to be received directly and efficiently.

Maria: Maria had cancer. Having to go through chemo and radiation treatments was absolutely terrifying for her. I had worked for years with patients undergoing treatments therefore, teaching Maria several stress reduction imageries was immensely helpful for her emotionally and mentally because she felt empowered to participate in the healing process.

A note on the compromised immune system

As far as healings go, anyone with a compromised immune system needs healings to maintain the chakra / auric field. And anyone undergoing surgery and invasive medical treatments like chemo will definitely regain strength more quickly after having several healings right after their procedures. The body's natural energy systems of these patients are so terribly disrupted that healings and all holistic supplemental remedies are absorbed by the body instantly.

The body is starving for life force. I think my most gratifying work has been in helping these patients. What seemed like magic to them is not. Eventually, clients learn this and, before you know it, they are telling their friends to take a deep breath, meditate, come to the yoga class, eat a banana (instead of that Twinkie), or to go to the park instead of the mall today.

Relax and get back in touch with the true nature of who you are by reuniting with the natural world. The natural world is the proper balance of electrons, atoms, cells and systems. Everything we are comprised of is in the natural world, above and below. What once seemed like magic or weird new–age practice is finally understood and innately remembered as common sense.

"New age" knowledge is not new. This knowledge has come down through thousands of years of practice by every culture in the world. Our ancestors did not have doctors, they had medicine men and women, shamans, healers. We already have this knowledge. It is simply a matter of remembering it. This is why the body responds so positively to it.

Don

Don, 47, had his leg amputated below the knee. He was experiencing "phantom pain" (the sensation that the severed limb is still attached and can be "felt").

This is a somewhat complex and multi-faceted cause of pain, primarily due to neuromuscular (brain-to-muscle and nerve pathway) memory and of an auric field holding the missing leg's energy pattern.

In this case, I focused the healing energy on the end of the stump. I used the 20 Chakra Technique (including Localized Polarity with Color using Blue and Green) on the stump and it relieved his condition fairly quickly. (The Auric field will eventually shrink to the new configuration of the limb.)

This effect was evidenced in a pair of Kirlian (aura) photographs. The first was taken of a maple leaf that was whole and the auric field held the shape and contour of the leaf. In the second photograph, the leaf had been cut in half. However, the auric field retained its original outline. In subsequent photographs, the auric field gradually shrank to conform to the new configuration of the leaf (i.e. cut in half)

In performing a healing, the healer is accelerating this process, thus possibly sparing the recipient months of pain and suffering while waiting for it to happen naturally. All holistic health work accelerates healing of any kind for body, mind and spirit.

Knowing your limitations

Alternatively, there have been clients whom I couldn't help. Every healer has a forte and limitations for whatever reason. For example, I can't seem to significantly help clients with back and spine problems. I don't know why, but I've finally accepted the fact and tell them so. I can help with pain reduction through hypnotherapy but that seems to be the extent of it. So, as in any profession, know your limitations and refer clients when necessary.

Lastly, trust your abilities. Share what you know! Let's all help our world, one person at a time. Think globally, act locally. As I heal, we all heal. As you heal, we all heal. And thank you because you matter!

Test: Healing with the Senses
(For Certification)

Requirements:

Please answer each question on a *separate sheet(s) of paper*. For certification purposes include the following:

- Your name
- Date you are completing this test
- Write/type out each question, then answer it.

Acupressure Points

1) How long do you press an acupressure point?

2) Which point aides asthma?

3) Which point aides fatigue?

4) Which point relieves headaches?

5) When do you never use this point?

Sound Frequency

1. How do sound frequencies aid in healing the body?

2. What is the difference between dissonant vibrations and consonance vibrations?

3. Give an example of a sound tool for each listed in question 2.

Chants

1. What are the benefits of chanting?

2. How do you think it works in relating to the energy fields of the body and in a room? (thought question)

Emotions and the Body

1. What emotions correlate with the heart chakra?

2. What emotions correlate with the liver?

3. If a client has a back problem, is that the masculine or feminine aspect of being?

4. What organs can be affected by stress in the feminine, front side of the body?

5. If a client is giving more than receiving in life, how would you know via the body?

6. Out of the 5 senses, which triggers memory most easily?

7. Which organ relates to the fear of living?

8. Which joints relate to the fear of moving forward?

Mind Body Dialogue

2) What are the 3 basic questions asked in this process?

3) What was your personal experience with the "Cellular Memory Imagery"?

Negative Extractions

1. When doubt exists as to which chakra is the source of the problem, name the chakra to use for this process.

2. After pulling out the root of the negative attachment (at the count of 3) and reciting "brief" affirmations, why is essential to allow a time of complete silence and physical distance for the client?

Chapter 10

Certification Procedures

"The heart of a human being is no different from the soul of heaven and earth. In your practice always keep in your thoughts the interaction of heaven and earth, water and fire, yin and yang."

MORIHEI UESHIBA

Certification Procedure

Requirements for Certification:

1. **Complete all tests (Please use the required format as instructed).**
   _____Chapter 2 Test 1: *Self Help Reflections*....................... pg 56
   _____Chapter 3 Test 2: *Energy Fields*............................... pg 71
   _____Chapter 3 Test 3: *Chakras*.......................................pg 81
   _____Chapter 4 Test 4: *Mind-Body Meditations*.................... pg 117
   _____Chapter 5 Test 5: *Preparation*................................pg 142
   _____Chapter 6 Test 6: *Healing Techniques*....................... pg 182
   _____Chapter 7 Test 7: *Healing with the Senses*.................. pg 244 -245

2. **Document 30 healings (using a variety of techniques), using the *"Client Log Sheet"* and *"Waiver & Assumption of Risk"* form signed by each of your 30 clients.**

3. **Complete 1 essay (at least one page in length) about your overall experience with the entire process.**

4. **Include the "Certification Submission form" on the next page. (Your written material can be emailed to ClaremontHealingUSA@gmail.com PDF format only or sent via postal service).**

5. **Book via PayPal: If you purchased the book via PayPal, we will need your name and date of purchase and/or transaction ID# from PayPal to verify the payment.**

6. **Submit Certificate Processing Fee: *$295***
   Include check or money order, payable to: Joanne Dinsmore or
   pay via PayPal through our website: ClaremontHealingUSA.com

Book evaluation: This is *not* mandatory for certification. We welcome your feedback. Please take a moment and let us know what you think about the book.

1. What did you like most about the book?
2. What could we improve on?
3. Is there any subject you would have liked more information on?
4. Is there any subject you would like to see covered in future editions?
5. Are the costs reasonable? For the book and/or certification?

Questions?
Contact: E-mail: ClaremontHealingUSA@gmail.com
www. ClaremontHealingUSA.com
(626) 802-0224

Certificate Submission Form:

You must contact us before sending in your submissions.
We do not return submitted materials. Please keep your own copies.

Please write your name *clearly*, as you want it to appear on your Certificates.

Your full name: _____

Address: _____

Phone:_____Email:_____

Because we have recently transitioned to an online business, please contact us for mailing instructions when you are ready to submit materials and apply for your certification.

Joanne Dinsmore

(626) 802-0224

claremonthealingusa@gmail.com

Are you interested in becoming a Certified Healing Practitioner Instructor (HPI) for this HP Program?
Yes____   No ____

Are you interested in hosting a workshop on any topics in this manual?
Yes____   No ____

When will I get my Certificates and HP/HHC bonus information pack?
Once you have submitted your fee and documentation listed above, you will receive your Certificates as a *Healing Arts Practitioner* and *Holistic Health Consultant including the bonus pack within 4-6 weeks* mailed via USPS. Any corrections from your submitted tests will be included.

The HP/HHC bonus information pack may be sent electronically in PDF format if you prefer. Please specify when submitting your certification fee.

www. ClaremontHealingUSA.com

Visit our Website for: Certifications, products, classes, calendar of local events and services offered.

Congratulations!

I hope I've served you well.
Brightest Blessings on your Journey

Joanne

Healing Arts Practitioner, Holistic Health Consultant Certificates & *Bonus Pack Details*

Two Professional Certificates as a: Healing Arts Practitioner and Holistic Health Consultant.

What's in the Bonus Pack?

- **The Claremont Healing Arts Center USA *Code of Ethics* Certificate**
  Including your name, the Claremont Healing Arts Center Seal and the Director's signature. Instills client's confidence in your professional integrity as a Healing Practitioner.

- **A document of subjects completed in this 300-hour HP/HHC certificate course.**

Starting your practice:
- **Client Information Sheet**
- **Initial Client Assessment (Body, Mind, Emotion & Spirit)**
- **Waiver & Assumption of Risk form**
- **Client Log Sheet**
- **The Healing Cheat Sheet**
- **Holistic Health Referrals form**

Starting Your Own Business:
- **How to Build Your Business from Scratch**
- **Bridging the Gap from Beginner to Pro**
- **Licensing Your Business (Going Professional)**
- **Mailing List Form (Gathering info for potential clients)**

Handouts for Your Clients:
- **How Vulnerable are you to stress?**
- **Life Stress Chart**
- **Adult Children of Alcoholics or Abuse-characteristics**
- **Characteristics of Co-Dependents**
- **The Wheel of Balance evaluation and more**

Note: If you wish to retain your submitted material, please make copies for yourself. We will only return to you any corrections made from your test questions.

The Healing Cheat Sheet

Preparing for the Client

1. *Light your altar candle* and recite your prayer. (For example: "Spirit, help me be the perfect conduit for my client's highest good.")

2. *Smudge the room* and yourself, clearing out any unwanted energies.

3. *Do your Chakra Imagery* and quiet meditation.

4. *Prepare the healing table* or area and the crystal layout if desired.

Part 1- Before the Healing

1. *Specific areas of concern:* Ask your client about their concerns while making notes in the Client Log Sheet.

2. *Do a "check-in":* on a scale of 1-10.

3. *Scan* the aura and chakras, paying special attention to the client's concerns noted before the session began.

4. *Smudge* around the client.

5. *Aromatherapy:* use "Relax" or "Sacred" oil. Put a drop in the client's palm. Have them rub their hands together and breathe in deeply a few times.

6. *Imagery*: Verbalize an appropriate one for the client.

Part 2- Performing the Healing

7. *Sit at the Crown* and channel an energy connection with Spirit.

8. *Healing technique-* Begin the chosen technique.

9. *Address specific areas* of concern.

10. *Add* appropriate options throughout the healing: reflexology, color, acupressure points, stones, sounds, chants, mind/body dialogue, cellular memory, breathing techniques, symbols, negative extractions (to be used at the end).

Compliments of The Claremont Healing Arts

Part 3- Closing

1. *Close:* Smudge, sweep and bubble.

2. *Scan:* re-assess aura and chakra.

3. **Aromatherapy**: use "Energy", 1 drop on your palm. Rub and wave over the client. Put one drop on client's palm and have them rub their hands together and breathe in deeply to wake up.

4. *Do another "check-in":* on a scale of 1-10.

Part 4- After

1. *Blow out the candle* on your altar with gratitude.

2. *Cleanse/Ground yourself* by washing your hands in water or rubbing them in rock salt or by sitting in nature to re-balance.

3. *Log the healing information* on the client's log sheet.

4. *Cleanse all stones and tools* used during the healing in water, salt, sun or earth.

JESUS PERFORMED MIRACLES, NOT BECAUSE HE BELIEVED HE COULD, BUT BECAUSE HE KNEW HE COULD. THAT IS WHY HE GAVE THANKS IN ADVANCE.
Conversations with God
Neal Donald Walsch

Client Log Sheet

Name:_____ Age:_____

Address:_____ _____
              (Street #/Name)   (City)

        _____ _____
              (State/Zip)   (Phone Number and Email)

. . . .

*Specific areas of concern:*_____

_____

_____

Date:_____   Check-in: *Before*:_____ *After*:_____

Scan observations *before*:_____

_____

Scan observations *after*:_____

_____

Healing Technique & Additions:_____

_____

Client's experience/comments:_____

_____

_____

Notes for future healing:_____

_____

_____

_____

_____

WAIVER AND ASSUMPTION OF RISK

I,_____, Customer, voluntarily sign this Waiver and Assumption of

Risk in favor of the Healing Practitioner and Holistic Health Consultant, _____
_____, in consideration for the opportunity to use the Healer's
facilities and/or the opportunity to receive instruction from the Healer or the Healer's employees
and/or to engage in the activities sponsored by the Healer, as follows:

I fully assume any risks involved as acceptable to me and I agree to use my best judgment in
undertaking these activities and to follow all safety instructions. I agree to consult my physician
before using any supplements, including herbs and aromas and before receiving any healings or other
services provided by the Healer.

I waive and release the Healer from any claim for personal injury, property damage, or death that
may arise from my use of the facilities or from my participation in any activities or instruction.

I am a competent adult, aged_____and I assume any risks of my own free will.

Dated:_____, 20 ____

_____
Signature of Customer

_____
Printed Name of Customer

_____
Address of Customer

_____
City and State of Customer

Recommended Reading & Resources

Books

Spiritual Healing
Scientific Validation of a Healing
Revolution
Daniel J. Benor, M.D.

Essential Oils
Susan Curtis

Homecoming
John Bradshaw

Between Heaven and Earth
A Guide to Chinese Medicine
Harriet Beinfield, L.Ac.

Hands of Light
Barbara Brennan

Healing Touch
A Resource for Healthcare Professionals
Dorthea Hover-Kramer, EdD, RN

Cell-Level Healing
Joyce Whiteley Hawkes Ph.D.

The Alchemist
Paulo Coelho

The Travelers Gift
Andy Andrews

The Secret
Rhonda Byrne

A New Earth
Eckhart Tolle

*The Complete Book of Essential
Oils & Aromatherapy*
Valarie Ann Worwood

The Celestine Prophecy
James Redfield

The Way of the Peaceful Warrior
Dan Millman

Staying Healthy with the Seasons
Elson M. Haas M.D.

Love is in the Earth
A Kaleidoscope of Crystals
Melody

*Traveling the Wyrd Path:
A Seeker's Map to Hands-On Spirituality*
Julie Bradshaw

The Body Electric
Electromagnetism And
The Foundation Of Life
Robert Becker, Gary Selden

Movies

The Secret

Directed by: Drew Heriot
Primetime Studios
DVD and streaming 2006

The Celestine Prophecy
Directed by: Armand Mastroianni
Celestine Films LLC
DVD 2006

What the Bleep Do We Know!?

Directed by: Betsy Chasse, Mark Vicente,
William Arntz
20 Century Fox
DVD 2005

Essential Oils, Bulk Herbs & Packaging

Starwest Botanicals - essential & carrier oils

www.starwestbotanicals.com

1-(800) 800-4372 Mon- Fri 8 AM – 5 PM (PST)
Rancho Cordova, California

. . . .

New Directions Aromatics - essential & carrier oils

www.newdirectionsaromatics.com

1-(800) 246-7817 Mon- Fri 9 AM – 5 PM (EST)

. . . .

E.D. Luce Packaging - bottles, droppers, jars etc.

www.essentialsupplies.com

1-(800) 246-7817 Mon- Fri 9 AM – 5 PM (EST)

. . . .

Mountain Rose Herbs - bulk herbs, press n seal tea bags, muslin bags etc.

www.mountainroseherbs.com

(800) 879-3337
Eugene, Oregon

Tuning Forks, Chimes & Accu Trigger

School for Inner Sound Therapy

www.ardenwilken.com
 (click on Tuning Forks to order online)

Contact Tel: +44 (0)208 891 3798
Middlesex, England Great Britain

. . . .

Song Pods
www.SongPods.com
(330) 401-5624
Jimm Song Pods
P.O. Box 9
Tippecanoe, OH 44699 US
Email: SongPods@Live.com

Accupoint
Pen Sparker
(Search online)

Crystals & Healing Stones

Jewel Tunnel Imports - wholesale crystals, stones, jewelry supplies etc.)

www.jeweltunnel.com

(626) 814-2257 Mon – Fri 9AM – 5PM (PST)
Baldwin Park, California
....

Annual Quartzsite Hobby, Craft & Gem Show

www.quartzsitervshow.com
(click on "craft show" and "general info")

Late January to early February

Show Location - 700 S. Central, Quartzsite, Arizona
....

Kacha Stones
Ethically mined crystals and stones dug out by hand, not blasted out

www.kachastones.com

Offer free international shipping (see website for details)
Newcastle Emlyn, Dyfed, Wales Great Britain

Becoming an Ordained Minister

Universal Life Church Monastery
Legal Ordained Minister Registration online (required for "hands on" healing in lieu of a massage license)

http://www.themonastery.org/

(206) 285-1086 -Monday -Friday, 9am and 4pm PST Seattle, WA

About the Author

Joanne Kain-Dinsmore

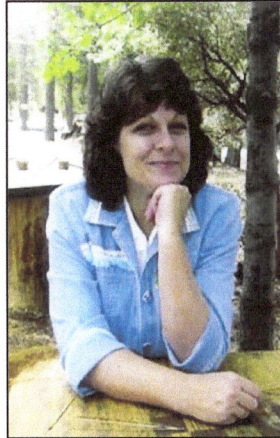

Joanne is the Executive Director and founder of the Claremont Healing Arts Center of America.

She is a Drug & Alcohol Counselor, specializing in Codependency and Inner child work after having interned at the John Bradshaw Center, Ingleside Hospital, CA. in 1992.

Her life-long interests and studies in natural medicine and healing arts led to a Holistic Health education program she taught at numerous locations, including Health Plans in So. Cal. In 1995, she designed the Healing Arts Practitioner Certification curriculum and has taught the course in her center to hundreds of students from all walks of life.

She continues her pursuit of knowledge in life-coaching, holistic health, hypnotherapy and Reiki. She is also author of *Still Eternal*: *the Petals and Thorns of a Lifetime*.

She lives in Southern California with her husband, Doug and their 3 furry kids: Apollo (the Pomeranian) and the cats, The Empress Sophie and Miss "T".

Parting words from Joanne

I wrote the following poem years ago when I, like you, first entered this road less traveled and at the point when I first recognized the transformations that were taking place within myself.

The positive changes in body, mind, emotions and spirit were so subtle and gradual that only in retrospect did I fully realize how far I had come.

I cherish my journey as a spiritual seeker and healer. I have healed many wounds, awakened my true self and have been blessed in the opportunities to guide others to do the same.

I sincerely hope that this book has inspired you to seek and find your True Path of healing and purpose. Life is a journey, not a destination. May your journey be as honest, true and blessed as it has been for me.

Gratefully,
Joanne

The Dawning

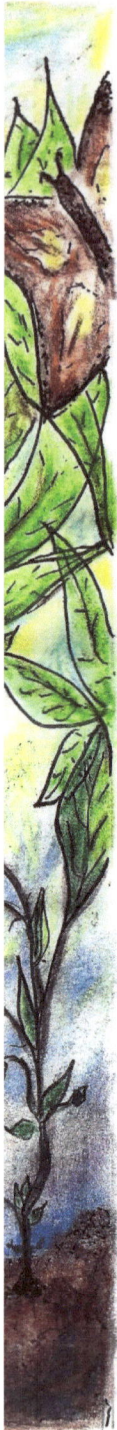

Sleepy cat ears
turn to blades of grass
stirred by the wind.

Pebbles loosen from an age-old cliff,
altering then what it has been.
Sometimes growth moves as graceful as that.

Just when I'm wondering what more there is,
the unseen sprouts another inch
under the hardened harvest.

Just when I breathe crimson leaves
of a waning season, a dayspring cloud
fills my head, softening through me,

washing sweet in changing me.
I feel the dawning like the morning sun
drapes upon a sleeping chill.

The dawning
of a changing rock,
despite myself,

unfurling something new.
A blossom soon,
unveiling color and core

and in wonder of it's own loveliness.
For there, within, I am born
another seed.

What more might I wonder after that?
Like the caterpillar
that sheds to wings

So humble
is the dawning
for so great the metamorphosis

By Joanne Dinsmore

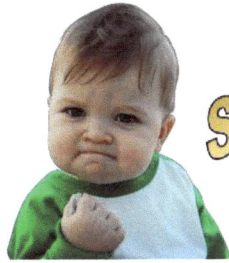

Success!

YES! You did it!

You reached the end of Volume 1

Now farther down the road… *VOLUME 2*

Traveling the Wyrd Path: A Seeker's Map for Hands-On Spirituality
by Julie Bradshaw

This little tyke above has to be Julie's clone!
Julie is a powerhouse of light, creativity, determination and humor (as will be evident when you pick up this book). There is much more to learn through her (3rd) eye and experiences.

Traveling the Wyrd Path: A Seeker's Map for Hands-On Spirituality is fun, and super informative. She will take you along her travels and training in Ireland, expounding more on the (Celtic) Shaman Path.

Other topics in her artistic manual include:

- More Stone Layouts

- The Medicine Wheel

- Herbs, teas and sachets

- Healing Tools and how to make your own

- Symbols from several cultures for healing and intention

- Developing your intuition

- The core practices of Shamanism with the Celtic culture applied

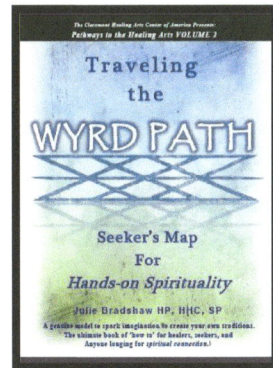

All of which will immensely add to your personal journey as a self-healer or a professional healer. Full of insight, her esoteric knowledge will inspire your creativity, reminding you what it is to "wonder" while you wander down the healing path.

She shares many anecdotes and stories describing both the inner and outer challenges she faced and the gifts she received from them. ENJOY!

www.ingramcontent.com/pod-product-compliance
Lightning Source LLC
Chambersburg PA
CBHW061134030426

42334CB00003B/37